A Practical Guide to Ultrasound in Obstetrics and Gynecology

Eric E. Sauerbrei, B.S., M.S., M.D., F.R.C.P.(C.)
Associate Professor of Radiology

Khanh T. Nguyen, M.S., M.D., F.R.C.P.(C.)
Assistant Professor of Radiology

Robert L. Nolan, B.S., M.D., F.R.C.P.(C.)
Assistant Professor of Radiology

*Queen's University
Kingston General Hospital
Kingston, Ontario K7L 2V7*

Raven Press ✍ New York

Raven Press, 1185 Avenue of the Americas, New York, New York 10036

Made in the United States of America

Library of Congress Cataloging-in-Publication Data
Sauerbrei, Eric E.
  A. practical guide to ultrasound in obstetrics and gynecology.

  Includes bibliographies and index.
    1. Diagnosis, Ultrasonic.   2. Generative organs, Female—Diseases
—Diagnosis.   3. Ultrasonics in obstetrics. I. Nguyen, Khanh T. II.
Nolan, Robert L. (Robert Louis) III. Title. [DNLM: 1. Fetal Diseases—
diagnosis.   2. Genital Diseases, Female—diagnosis.
3. Hysterosalpingography—methods.   4. Pregnancy Complications—
diagnosis.   5. Ultrasonic Diagnosis—methods. WQ 240 S255p]
  RG107.5.U4S27 1987   618.2'07543   86-28009
  ISBN 0-88167-268-8

9 8 7 6 5 4 3 2

A PRACTICAL GUIDE TO ULTRASOUND
IN OBSTETRICS AND GYNECOLOGY

This book is dedicated to
Tyler
Peter

Daphne
Jade

Erin
Kathryn
Lisa

Preface

The purpose of this short guide is to portray the ultrasound appearance of the normal structures in obstetrics and gynecology and the abnormalities most commonly found in our clinical practice. In so doing we hope to cover most entities that will be encountered in the general practice of ultrasound in obstetrics and gynecology.

This is not meant to be a complete text of this large subject; therefore, less common lesions and variants of normal, as well as complete discussions on each topic, are not included. We have instead chosen to emphasize the scan appearance of various entities and to provide brief, pertinent, and clinically useful text to complement the scans. Of necessity, the material and ideas in the book reflect the authors' clinical experiences and biases; we feel, however, that it presents a fair reflection of common ultrasound practice in obstetrics and gynecology.

In the chapter on fetal measurements and calculations and in the Appendix, we have included the fetal measurements that we routinely use, and we have presented abbreviated tables, graphs, and simple computer programs that we utilize to derive clinically useful parameters, such as fetal weight estimations. Again, the goal is to provide only the measurements and calculations that we find useful on a daily basis. For those measurements and calculations that we use rarely, other references must be consulted.

This book will be especially helpful to general radiologists, obstetricians, and gynecologists.

ERIC E. SAUERBREI
KHANH T. NGUYEN
ROBERT L. NOLAN

Acknowledgments

The most important feature of this guide is the ultrasound scan, which should portray clearly the normal structure or the lesion considered. We are fortunate to work with excellent sonographers who provided many of the examples included in this guide: Cathy Marshall, A.R.D.M.S.; Rhonda Emmons, A.R.D.M.S.; Florine Robichaud, A.R.D.M.S., Leslie Wilberforce, A.R.D.M.S.; and Maureen O'Connor, A.R.D.M.S..

Typing numerous drafts and preparing the format for chapters are long and demanding tasks, and for performing these accurately and with good cheer, we thank Yvonne DeRoche.

We would like to thank Mr. Charlie Pearson for a fine job of photographing the prints and Mr. Stan Morton for the artwork.

For providing clinical assistance and scan material, we would like to acknowledge and thank the following: the Department of Obstetrics and Gynecology at Kingston General Hospital, Queen's University (especially Dr. Robert L. Reid, Dr. Paul MacKenzie, and Dr. Mike McGrath); the Department of Pathology of Kingston General Hospital, Queen's University (especially Dr. Howard Steele and Dr. Allan Fletcher); Dr. Ants Toi at Toronto General Hospital, Department of Radiology; Dr. John Flatman and Dr. Ian Leggett at St. Mary's General Hospital, Timmins, Ontario.

We would like to give special thanks to the radiologists at the Kingston General Hospital, Queen's University for their support in this project.

Contents

Chapter 1

INDICATIONS FOR ULTRASOUND DURING PREGNANCY

In 1984, the National Institutes of Health (NIH) sponsored a consensus development conference to assess the use of diagnostic ultrasound imaging during pregnancy. The conference was held after a year of preparation by the panel that included input from many sources. One of several questions posed to the panel was the following: Based on the available evidence, what are the appropriate indications for, and limitations on, the use of ultrasound in obstetrics today? The following is the consensus statement in response to this question:

From the body of information reviewed, taking into account the available bioeffects literature, data on clinical efficacy, and with concern for psychosocial, economic, and legal/ethical issues, *it is the consensus of the panel that ultrasound examination in pregnancy should be performed for a specific medical indication.* The data on clinical efficacy and safety do not allow a recommendation for routine screening at this time.

Ultrasound examinations performed solely to satisfy the family's desire to know the fetal sex, to view the fetus, or to obtain a picture of the fetus should be discouraged. In addition, visualization of the fetus solely for educational or commercial demonstrations without medical benefit to the patient should not be performed.

Prior to an ultrasound examination, patients should be informed of the clinical indication for ultrasound, specific benefit, potential risk, and alternatives, if any. In addition, the patient should be supplied with information about the exposure time and intensity, if requested. A written form may expedite this process in some cases.

Patient access to educational materials regarding ultrasound is strongly encouraged. All settings in which these examinations are conducted should assure patients' dignity and privacy.

Given that the full potential of diagnostic ultrasound imaging is critically dependent on examiner training and experience, the panel recommends minimum training requirements and uniform credentialing for all physicians and sonographers performing ultrasound examinations. All health care providers who use this modality should demonstrate adequate knowledge of the basic physical principles of ultrasound, equipment, recordkeeping requirements, indications and safety.

The panel further provided a list of 28 clinical situations in which ultrasound could be of benefit. These are beyond the scope of this book and are available in NIH Publication No. 84-667 entitled *Diagnostic Ultrasound Imaging in Pregnancy.*[1]

It is worth emphasizing that the opinion of the panel with regard to routine ultrasound scanning in obstetrics may be summarized by the statement by Mortimer B. Lipsett, M.D., Director, National Institute of Child Health and Human Development, in the preface to the report:

> I would like to point out that the panel's decision not to endorse routine ultrasound screening of pregnant women is based on the observation that there is not enough evidence that routine screening benefits either the mother or the fetus and is not based on any evidence of harm or damage to either mother or fetus.

---

[1]Report of a consensus development conference sponsored by the National Institute of Child Health and Human Development, the Office of Medical Applications of Research, the Division of Research Resources, and the Food and Drug Administration, Feb. 6–8, 1984, NIH, Bethesda, Maryland.

Chapter 2

GUIDELINES FOR OBSTETRICAL ULTRASOUND EXAMINATIONS

The following guidelines are excerpted from a publication from The American College of Radiology entitled *Policy Statement. Antepartum Obstetrical Ultrasound Examination Guidelines*.

Equipment

These studies should be conducted with real-time, or a combination of real-time and static scanners, but never solely with a static scanner. A transducer of appropriate frequency (in the 3–5 MHz range) should be used.

Documentation

Adequate documentation of the study is essential for high-quality patient care. This should include a permanent record of the ultrasound images with appropriate labeling.

Whenever possible, an attempt should be made to demonstrate the measurement parameters and anatomical findings proposed below.

A written report of the ultrasound findings should be included in the patient's medical record. The images should be labeled with the examination date, patient identification, and image orientation.

Guidelines for First Trimester

1. The location of the gestational sac should be documented. The embryo should be identified and the crown–rump length recorded.
2. Presence or absence of fetal life should be reported.

Comment: Real-time observation is critical in this diagnosis. It should be noted that cardiac activity may not be visible prior to 7 weeks as determined by crown–rump length. Thus, confirmation of fetal life may require follow-up evaluation.

3. Fetal number should be documented.
4. Evaluation of the uterus (including cervix) and adnexal structures should be performed.

Guidelines for Second and Third Trimesters

1. Fetal life, number, and presentation should be documented.

   Comment: Abnormal heart rate and/or rhythm should be reported. Multiple pregnancies require the reporting of additional information: placental number, sac number, and comparison of fetal size.

2. An estimate of the amount of amniotic fluid (increased, decreased, normal) should be reported.

3. The placental location should be recorded and its relationship to the internal cervical os determined.

4. Assessment of gestational age in the second and third trimester should be accomplished using at least two of the following parameters: (a) biparietal diameter, (b) head circumference, (c) femur length, and (d) abdominal circumference. If previous studies have been done, an estimate of the appropriateness of interval growth should be given.

   a. *Biparietal diameter* at a standard reference level should be measured and recorded and should include the cavum septi pellucidi, the thalamus, or the cerebral peduncles to confirm that the appropriate level was selected.

   b. *Head circumference* is measured at the same level as the biparietal diameter.

   c. *Femur length* should be measured routinely and recorded after the twelfth week of gestation.

   d. *Abdominal circumference* should be determined at the level of the junction of the umbilical vein and portal sinus.

5. Evaluation of the uterus (including cervix) and adnexal structures should be performed.

6. The study should include an attempt to demonstrate but not necessarily be limited to the following fetal anatomy: cerebral ventricles, spine, stomach, urinary bladder, umbilical cord insertion site, and renal region. Suspected abnormalities may require a specialized evaluation.

Chapter 3

NORMAL PELVIC ANATOMY

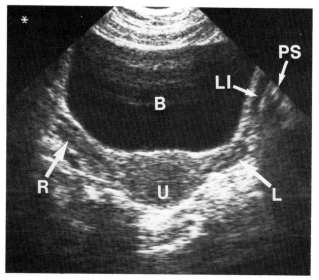

1. Transverse scan: (B) urinary bladder; (U) uterus; (R) right ovary; (L) left ovary; (LI) left iliac vessel; (PS) Iliopsoas muscle.

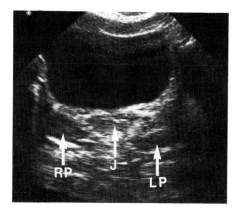

2. Transverse scan: (J) junction of cervix and vagina; (RP) right piriformis muscle; (LP) left piriformis muscle.

Chapter 4

THE NONGRAVID UTERUS

The Neonatal Uterus

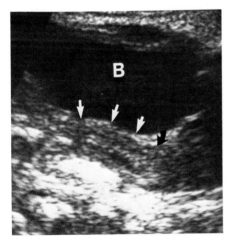

3. Sagittal scan of the uterus; infant, age 2 days: (B) bladder; (*arrows*) uterus. The uterus is difficult to appreciate because it is retroflexed and rectal contents posterior to the uterus obscure the posterior border.

4. Sagittal scan of the uterus; same infant, age 1 month: (B) bladder; (*arrows*) uterus. Note the central hyperechoic zone corresponding to the endometrial lining.

Maternal hormonal stimulation of the fetal uterus results in a relatively large uterus in the early neonatal period. At this stage, the uterine body is larger than the cervix. As the effect of maternal hormonal stimulation dissipates, the uterine size decreases and gradually develops into the infantile or premenarchal pattern. At this stage, the body is smaller than the cervix.

Since the neonatal uterus may be quite large and not resemble the usual pattern of uterine anatomy, a pelvic mass in a neonate should be interpreted cautiously unless a normal uterus is also visualized.

The Premenarchal Uterus

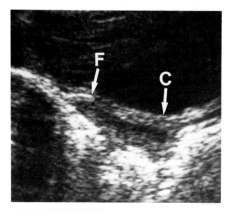

5. Sagittal scan of uterus; age 3 years: (C) cervix; (F) fundus.

The uterus in the premenarchal age group is small in size, with the body smaller in diameter than the cervix. There is gradual growth throughout childhood. An endometrial line is often visualized in the neonatal and premenarchal period.

The Postmenarchal Uterus

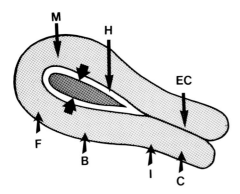

6. Diagram of sagittal axis of the uterus: (F) fundus; (B) body; (I) isthmus; (C) cervix; (EC) endocervical canal; (H) halo; (M) myometrium; (*arrowheads*) *T*, representing two layers of endometrium.

Anatomically, the uterus is divided into several segments. The fundus is the portion of the uterus above the orifices of the fallopian tubes. The body is the expanded portion consisting of the bulk of the organ. The isthmus is the slightly constricted lower portion separating the body from the cervix. The endocervical canal runs through the cervix into the endometrial cavity. The body is larger in diameter than the cervix. The nulliparous uterus is smaller than the parous uterus. It is usually *anteverted* (tilted anteriorly at a fulcrum point at the cervicovaginal junction); however, it may be *anteflexed* (flexed anteriorly at a fulcrum point at the isthmus).

The normal myometrium has a homogeneous texture. The hypoechoic halo surrounding the endometrium represents the inner one-eighth of the myometrium, containing submucosal vascular plexuses.

The endometrium is taken to be the hyperechoic line or band in the central portion of the uterus. The total thickness of the endometrium T represents two layers of endometrium. Therefore, $t = T/2$, where t is the single layer thickness.

The Postmenarchal Uterus (*contd.*)

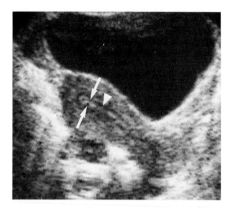

7. Proliferative (follicular) phase; sagittal scan of the uterus: (*arrows*) *T*, representing two layers of endometrium; (*arrowhead*) halo.

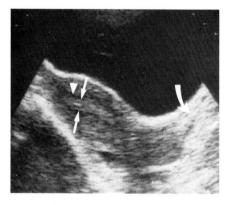

8. Secretory (luteal) phase; sagittal scan of the uterus: (*arrows*) *T*; (*arrowhead*) halo; (*curved arrow*) vaginal mucosa.

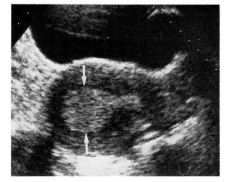

9. Sagittal scan of a uterus with a thick but normal endometrium in the secretory phase: (*arrows*) total endometrial thickness, *T*. *T* measures 3.4 cm at the location indicated.

The Postmenarchal Uterus (*contd.*)

In the *proliferative (follicular) phase,* the endometrium appears as a thin line or relatively thin hyperechoic band. This gradually thickens in the later proliferative phase.

In the *secretory (luteal) phase,* the endometrium appears as a relatively thick hyperechoic band.

The normal endometrial thickness varies greatly during the menstrual cycle and from one patient to another. It is unusual for the endometrial thickness T to be greater than 1.5 cm; however, it is occasionally much thicker. Most patients with a thick endometrium prior to menopause will be normal. The endometrial thickness T is an unreliable indicator of disease prior to menopause.

During the menstrual phase, a small amount of fluid may be present in the endometrial cavity between the layers of the endometrium t. The endometrium reverts to the appearance of the proliferative phase after menstruation.

The *vagina* is caudal to the bladder angle and cervix. The *vaginal mucosa* appears as a relatively thin hyperechoic line between the linear vesicovaginal septum anteriorly and the rectovaginal septum posteriorly.

The Postmenopausal Uterus

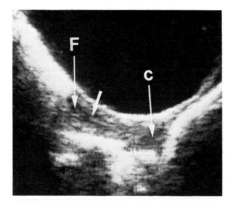

10. Sagittal scan of the uterus: (C) cervix; (F) fundus; (*arrow*) endometrium *T*.

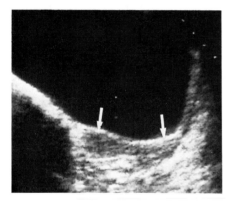

11. Sagittal scan of an atrophic uterus: (*arrows*) fundus and cervix of an atrophic uterus. Note that an endometrial line is not present.

The size of the postmenopausal uterus is variable. Reliable measurements are not available. There is gradual atrophy after menopause. The uterus may atrophy to the size of an infantile uterus and occasionally cannot be demonstrated.

The thin hypoechoic zone may be visualized around a thin hyperechoic endometrium. Reliable measurements for endometrial thickness *T* are not available; however, any endometrial thickness $T \geq 5$ mm is suspicious for pathology. We do not usually see the endometrium in the atrophic uterus.

The uterus may remain relatively large, with a prominent endometrium as a result of exogenous hormonal stimulation (estrogens).

Normal Variants of the Uterus

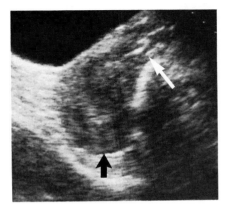

12. Sagittal scan of a retroverted uterus: (*white arrows*) cervix; (*black arrow*) fundus.

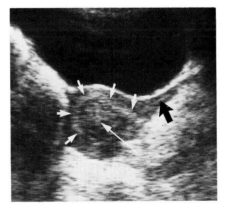

13. Sagittal scan of a retroflexed uterus: (*arrows*) endometrial cavity of a markedly retroflexed uterus; (*long arrow*) fulcrum point; (*black arrow*) vaginal mucosa.

These represent variations in position: the *retroverted uterus* is tilted posteriorly with a fulcrum point at the cervico-vaginal junction; the *retroflexed uterus* is flexed posteriorly with a fulcrum point at the isthmus of the uterus.

The retroverted/retroflexed uterus may show hypoechoic "dropout" at the fundus because of acoustic attenuation. This should not be misinterpreted as a mass (leiomyoma). A leiomyoma at this location may be difficult to diagnose for the same reason.

Normal Variants of the Uterus (*contd.*)

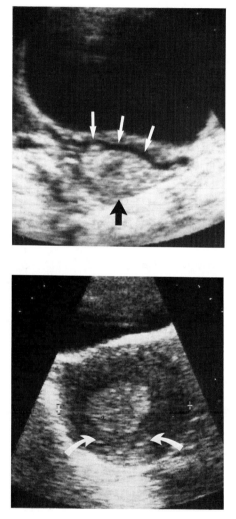

14. Transverse scan of the uterus; arcuate veins: (*white arrows*) arcuate vein; (*black arrow*) uterus.

15. Transverse scan of the uterus; enhancement posterior to the endometrium: (*curved arrows*) enhancement.

Arcuate arteries and veins run transversely through the anterior and posterior myometrium of the isthmus and body of the uterus. The arcuate veins are occasionally visualized in these locations.

Acoustic enhancement posterior to the endometrium and edge refraction at the margins of the endometrium are normal findings. These are usually seen in the secretory phase.

Uterine Appearance and Dimensions[a]

Uterine stage	Gross features	Length (cm ± SD)	Width of body (cm ± SD)	AP diameter of body (cm ± SD)	Approximate volume (cc ± SD)
Neonatal	Body > cervix	3.4 ±0.65	1.26 ±0.29	—	—
Premenarchal					
<7 years	Body < cervix	3.3 ±0.4	0.7 ±0.5	0.7 ±0.3	2.0 ±1.6
>7 years	Body > cervix Measurements gradually increase with age	3.6-5.4[b] ±1.0	0.8-1.5[b] ±0.5	0.9-1.7[b] ±0.5	3-16[b] ±1.5-9.0
Postmenarchal					
Nulliparous	Body > cervix	8.1 ±0.8	5.1 ±2.8	4.3 ±1.1	90 ±22
Parous	Body > cervix	Tends to be larger than nulliparous uterus by approximately 1 cm in each axis; no reliable measurements available			
Postmenopausal	Gradual atrophy after menopause	No reliable measurements available			

[a]Length is measured from cervix to fundus; width is measured at greatest width; AP is measured at greatest AP dimension in body; approximate volume is calculated by a modified formula for the volume of a prolate ellipsoid

$$V = \frac{4}{3}\pi \times \frac{1}{2}L \times \frac{1}{2}W \times \frac{1}{2}D$$

or by a simplified formula $V = 0.523 \times L \times W \times D$.

[b]Expressed as a range because of the wide range of biologic variation from age 7 years to menarche.

Congenital Disorders of the Uterus: Bicornuate Uterus

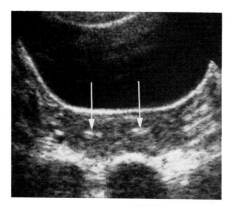

16. Transverse scan of the uterus; bicornuate uterus: (*arrows*) separate endometrial cavities.

Congenital disorders may be isolated or may occur in association with renal or anorectal anomalies. There is a high incidence of genital anomalies associated with unilateral renal agenesis.

Varying degrees of uterine duplication may occur. The bicornuate uterus has two endometrial cavities that join caudally. They are separated by myometrium in the body but usually not at the fundus. One cornu may be hypoplastic; the other cornu may simulate a "normal" uterus with deviated fundus.

Congenital Disorders of the Uterus: Uterus Didelphys

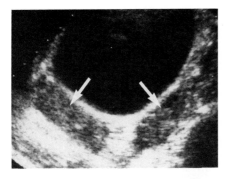

17. Transverse scan through the fundi; uterus didelphys: (*arrows*) separate endometrial cavities with separate fundi.

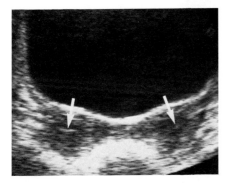

18. Transverse scan through the fundi; uterus didelphys: (*arrows*) separate endometrial cavities with joined fundi.

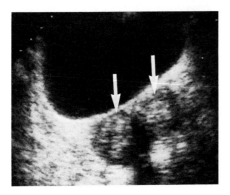

19. Transverse scan through the fused cervices of a uterus didelphys; (*arrows*) fused left and right cervices.

Uterus didelphys represents a double uterus with separate uterine bodies. These are usually fused at the cervix. Two external os are present. There may be a single or double vagina. The spectrum of findings in this entity is illustrated above.

Congenital Disorders of the Uterus: Hypoplastic Uterus

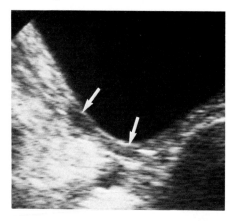

20. Sagittal scan of a hypoplastic uterus; primary ovarian failure, age 18 years: (*arrows*) uterus.

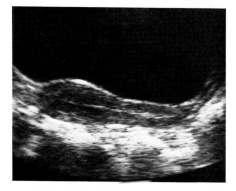

21. Sagittal scan of the uterus after 4 months of estrogen therapy in the same patient. The uterus has increased in size and has a postmenarchal appearance. The uterus has increased in length from 3 cm to 9 cm.

The hypoplastic uterus has a premenarchal pattern with decreased size. The endometrium may be seen in the larger uteri but not in very small ones. It is usually secondary to hypothalamic or pituitary hypofunction. Less frequently, it is the result of diethylstilbestrol exposure *in utero,* primary ovarian failure, and Turner's syndrome. Turner's syndrome also results in small ovaries.

The uterus is *aplastic* (completely absent) in the testicular feminization syndrome.

Uterine Masses: Leiomyoma(s) (Fibroids)

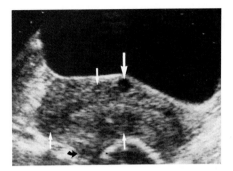

22. Sagittal scan of the uterus: (*large arrow*) small mass; (*small arrows*) inhomogeneous texture; (*black arrows*) contour change.

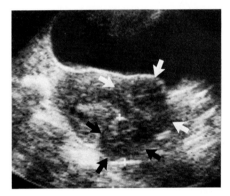

23. Transverse scan of the uterus: (*arrows*) two separate solid masses that give a lobulated contour to the uterus.

Leiomyomas (fibroids) are very common benign muscle tumors. They develop in approximately 25% of women during active reproductive life. Anatomically, they arise anywhere in the myometrium and, less frequently, from the broad ligament.

Small lesions are commonly missed. An inhomogenous texture of the myometrium without focal lesions may be seen with multiple small lesions.

The uterus is enlarged in approximately two-thirds of cases. A lobulated contour of the uterus is the most common sign. Subtle contour changes at the interface between the uterus and bladder are an early sign. The masses vary in size from small to very large.

Uterine Masses: Leiomyoma(s) (Fibroids) (*contd.*)

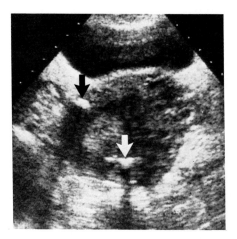

24. Transverse scan of the uterus; calcified leiomyomas in myometrium: (*arrows*) calcified foci within myometrium. Also note the inhomogeneous texture of the myometrium.

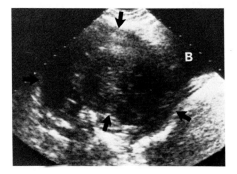

25. Sagittal scan of the uterus: (*arrows*) large leiomyoma; (B) bladder.   Normal anatomic structures could not be identified.

Masses are usually solid but are very rarely cystic due to degeneration. They are usually hypoechoic but are occasionally hyperechoic. Approximately 10% contain calcification, which causes focal acoustic attenuation.

Larger lesions may be inhomogenous due to degeneration. Very large lesions may distort the anatomy to the degree that we may not be able to determine the origin of the mass.

The endometrium may appear eccentrically located within the uterus due to mass effect.

Uterine Masses: Leiomyoma(s)   (Fibroids)   (*contd.*)

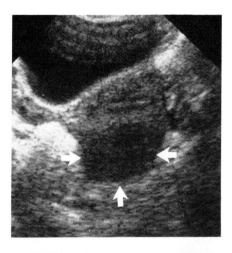

26. Transverse scan of the uterus; subserosal leiomyoma: (*arrows*) subserosal mass.

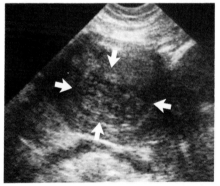

27. Sagittal scan of the uterus; submucosal leiomyoma: (*arrows*) submucosal mass that "fills" the endometrial cavity.

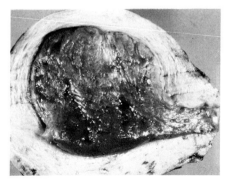

28. Pathological specimen of the submucosal leiomyoma shown in Fig. 27. There was red degeneration inside the leiomyoma.

Subserosal, pedunculated, or broad-ligament leiomyomas may simulate an adnexal mass. Submucosal leiomyomas may simulate an endometrial lesion or obstructed uterus.

Uterine Masses: Leiomyosarcoma

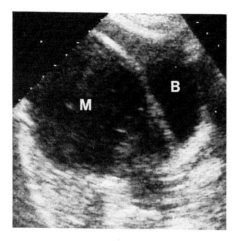

29. Sagittal scan of the uterus; leiomyosarcoma: (B) bladder; (M) large solid mass.

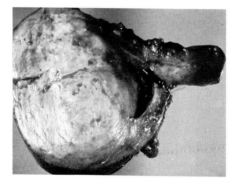

30. Pathological specimen of the leiomyosarcoma.

Leiomyosarcoma is a rare malignant tumor of the myometrium. It has the same ultrasound features as a leiomyoma. These entities cannot be differentiated on the basis of ultrasound appearance.

It usually presents as a solid mass or large lobulated uterus. The only ultrasound clue to the correct diagnosis may be a rapid increase in the size of a uterine mass or if there is postmenopausal bleeding associated with a mass.

Other pathological entities rarely present as a mass demonstrated on ultrasound. Rhabdomyosarcoma is a rare tumor in the pediatric age group. Carcinoma of the cervix is rarely diagnosed on ultrasound. It may present as a lower uterine segment mass or as an obstructed uterus. Rarely does lymphoma involve the uterus.

Uterine Masses: Nabothian Cyst

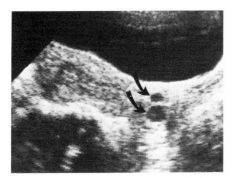

31. Sagittal scan of the uterus: (*arrows*) cysts in the cervix. Note the posterior acoustic enhancement.

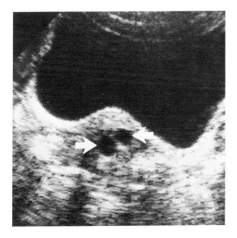

32. Transverse scan of the cervix: (*arrows*) cysts in the cervix.

Nabothian cysts are a gross manifestation of one of the features of chronic cervicitis. They represent cystic dilatation of the endocervical glands caused by inflammatory stenosis of their outlets. They are of no clinical significance.

Cysts can occur along the margin of the cervix or within the endocervical canal.

The Abnormal Endometrium

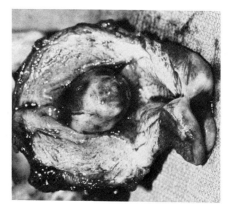

33. Sagittal scan of the uterus; polypoid lesion of the endometrium: (*arrows*) mass within the endometrial cavity.

34. Pathological specimen of the polypoid lesion.

Submucosal pedunculated leiomyomas and endometrial polyps may appear as a hypoechoic "mass" in the endometrium. Endometrial polyps are benign sessile lesions of the endometrium that occur most commonly around the menopause and cause abnormal uterine bleeding. These lesions can be demonstrated prior to menopause.

Prior to menopause, most patients with a thick endometrium will be normal; however, exogenous hormonal stimulation (estrogens) or adenomatous hyperplasia of the endometrium can cause a thick endometrium that is indistinguishable from the normal endometrium. Endometrial hyperplasia is associated with an increased risk of endometrial carcinoma.

We should be very cautious in interpreting an abnormal endometrium in the premenopausal uterus.

The Abnormal Endometrium (*contd.*)

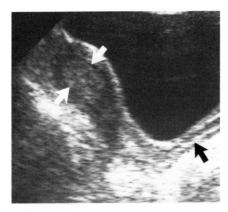

35. Sagittal scan of the uterus; exogenous hormonal stimulation, age 18 years: (*white arrows*) endometrium *T* measures 1.8 cm; (*black arrow*) vaginal mucosa.

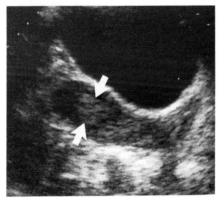

36. Sagittal scan of the uterus; endometrial carcinoma postmenopausal patient: (*arrows*) thickened endometrium; *T* measures 1.9 cm.

Reliable measurements for endometrial thickness T for the perimenopausal and postmenopausal uterus are *not* available. We would expect gradual atrophy of the endometrium during the perimenopausal period. We should, therefore, be cautious in our interpretation of the endometrial pattern in the perimenopausal period.

In the postmenopausal period, an endometrial thickness $T \geq 5$ mm is highly suspicious for pathology. A thickened endometrium can be caused by the following:

1. *Carcinoma of the endometrium* usually occurs in postmenopausal women. A thick endometrium in a patient with postmenopausal bleeding is very suggestive of this diagnosis. Occasionally, fluid will be seen in the endometrial cavity. When advanced, the body of the uterus may have an irregular contour.

2. *Cystic hyperplasia of the endometrium* occurs in the perimenopausal age groups and is the result of relative or absolute hyperestrinism. If found before puberty or after menopause, it strongly suggests a functioning ovarian tumor or adrenal cortical hyperfunction.

3. *Hyperechoic hematometra* may simulate a thickened endometrium.

The Abnormal Endometrium (*contd.*)

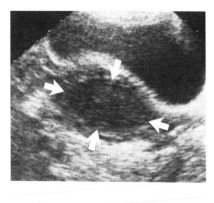

37. Sagittal scan of the uterus; endometrial carcinoma, post-menopausal patient: (*arrows*) fluid-filled endometrial cavity.

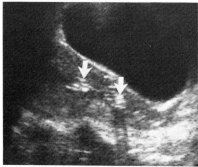

38. Sagittal scan of the uterus; pyometrium: (*arrows*) hyperechoic foci with acoustic attenuation due to gas in the endometrial cavity.

In the normal postmenarchal uterus, a small amount of fluid may be seen within the endometrial cavity during menses. In the premenarchal or postmenopausal uterus, fluid within the endometrial cavity usually indicates pathology.

Hydrometra/hematometra is the accumulation of secretions or blood within the endometrial cavity. *Hydrometrocolpos/hematometrocolpos* is the accumulation of secretions or blood within the vagina and endometrial cavity. The location of obstruction is determined by the fluid distribution. The etiology is usually congenital in premenarchal women and includes vaginal agenesis, transverse vaginal septum, and imperforate hymen. In older women, the cause is usually vaginal or cervical stenosis. Carcinoma of the endometrium and of the cervix should be excluded in the appropriate age groups.

An echogenic hematometra can simulate a thickened endometrium, but it actually represents blood within the endometrial cavity.

Pyometrium is rare. It may occur after sexual abuse, postoperatively, or with endometritis. Fluid in the endometrial cavity may be the only sign. Acoustic attenuation due to gas is highly suggestive of the diagnosis.

The Postpartum Uterus

39. Sagittal scan of the uterus; normal endometrial cavity, 5 days postpartum: (*small arrows*) normal endometrial cavity; (*large arrow*) small hyperechoic bladder-flap hematoma.

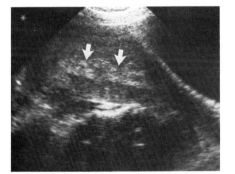

40. Sagittal scan of the uterus; retained placental tissue, 1 day postpartum: (*arrows*) hyperechoic tissue within the endometrial cavity.

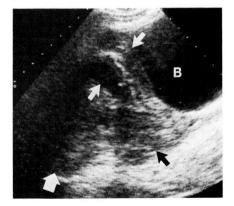

41. Sagittal scan of the uterus; bladder-flap hematoma: (*small black arrow*) cervix; (*large arrow*) fundus; (*small arrows*) mass having hypoechoic and hyperechoic features; (B) bladder.

The Postpartum Uterus (*contd.*)

The normal postpartum uterus may be quite large, depending on the time since delivery. Fluid is commonly seen within the endometrial cavity in the first postpartum week. There is a gradual decrease in size of the uterus, with regression to normal size within 2 to 3 months.

Retained products of conception (placental tissue) usually appears as a dense hyperechoic mass in the endometrial cavity.

A bladder flap hematoma occurs after a lower uterine transverse cesarean section. The hematoma is seen as a mass located between the bladder and the anterior aspect of the lower uterine segment. It may be hypoechoic, isoechoic, or hyperechoic. It may be inseparable from the anterior uterine wall. Bright echoes with posterior acoustic attenuation usually indicate an infected hematoma. Otherwise, we cannot differentiate among a hematoma, infected hematoma, and an abscess.

Intrauterine Contraceptive Devices: Normal

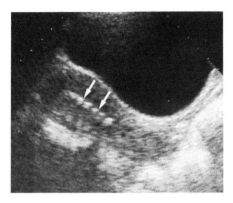

42. Sagittal scan of the uterus. A Lippe's loop is indicated by five interrupted hyperechoic lines with posterior acoustic attenuation: (*arrows*) Lippe's loop within the endometrial cavity.

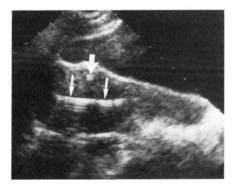

43. Sagittal scan of the uterus. A copper-T or copper-7 is indicated by entry–exit echos (*parallel lines*), ring-down artifact, and posterior acoustic attenuation: (*small arrows*) copper-T in the endometrial cavity; (*large arrow*) IUCD within the myometrium.

Intrauterine contraceptive devices (IUCDs) are a common form of birth control. We must be able to identify, localize, and detect complications associated with IUCDs.

The Lippe's loop is occasionally seen, and it is composed of polyethylene. A copper-7 or copper-T is commonly used and has fine copper wire wound around the proximal limbs.

The normal position for all IUCDs is high within the endometrial cavity of the body of the uterus.

A normally placed IUCD may be difficult to identify in the late secretory phase, due to prominent endometrial echoes. A normally placed IUCD may appear eccentrically placed with uterine leiomyomas, with a retroverted or retroflexed uterus, or with associated early pregnancy. IUCDs are difficult to identify in the retroverted or retroflexed uterus.

The Malpositioned IUCD

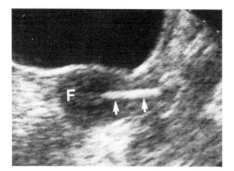

44. Type 1 malposition: (*arrows*) IUCD located low in the endometrial cavity and endocervical canal; (F) fundus.

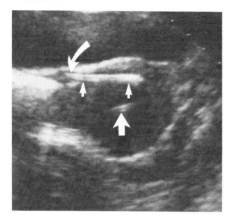

45. Type 2–3 malposition with adhesions to the transverse colon: (*small arrows*) IUCD in the myometrium; (*curved arrow*) IUCD perforating through the myometrium into the peritoneal cavity; (*large arrow*) another IUCD within the endometrial cavity. Note the entry-exit echoes.

The following classification of malpositioned IUCDs is based on anatomic location: type 1, endometrial; type 2, myometrial; type 3, peritoneal:

Type 1	Low in endometrial cavity and/or endocervical canal
Type 1–2	Endometrial + myometrial
Type 1–2–3	Endometrial + myometrial + peritoneal
Type 2	Myometrial
Type 2–3	Myometrial + peritoneal
Type 3	Intraperitoneal or retroperitoneal

Indications for Ultrasound in IUCDs

1. Certain situations predispose to malposition of an IUCD. Retroverted or retroflexed uterus, obesity, or postpartum status with soft myometrium all increase the risk of malposition. A traumatic or painful insertion would also suggest this possibility.

If the IUCD is not visualized on ultrasound, it may be due to spontaneous expulsion or, less commonly, perforation. Therefore, a plain radiograph of the abdomen is always indicated if the IUCD is not demonstrated in the normal position in the endometrial cavity.

Partial perforation, particularly type 1–2, remains a difficult and often missed diagnosis in spite of these investigative techniques. Intraperitoneal or retroperitoneal locations are usually not identified on ultrasound. Retroperitoneal placement as well as gradual erosion into adjacent structures, such as bowel or bladder, is rare.

2. Clinical history may suggest possible associated pelvic inflammatory disease, which occurs in 2% to 3% of patients. Ultrasound may show a mass or hydrosalpinx–pyosalpinx. Less severe forms of infection may show no abnormality.

3. Method failure with intrauterine pregnancy occurs in 2% to 5% of patients, depending on the type of IUCD. Ultrasound and a sensitive pregnancy test should be able to confirm the diagnosis as well as localize the intrauterine site of implantation. Ultrasound can also confirm the viability of the fetus, since there is a higher incidence of spontaneous abortion associated with the use of IUCDs.

Chapter 5

THE OVARIES AND ADNEXAE

The Reproductive Neurohormonal Axis

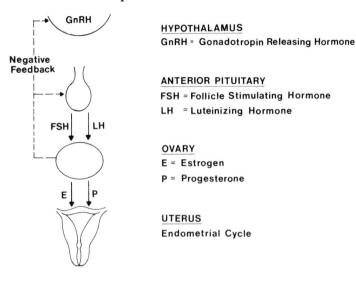

46

HYPOTHALAMUS
GnRH = Gonadotropin Releasing Hormone

ANTERIOR PITUITARY
FSH = Follicle Stimulating Hormone
LH = Luteinizing Hormone

OVARY
E = Estrogen
P = Progesterone

UTERUS
Endometrial Cycle

The hypothalamus secretes a polypeptide called gonadotropin-releasing hormone (GnRH), which induces the secretion of follicle-stimulating hormone (FSH) and luteinizing hormone (LH) from the anterior pituitary gland, and these hormones in turn cause the ovary to secrete estrogen and progesterone, which have a direct effect on the endometrium and myometrium of the uterus.

There is a negative feedback loop in this hormonal axis such that increasing levels of ovarian hormones cause decreasing secretions from the hypothalamus and pituitary.

Normal Hormonal Cycles and Ovulation

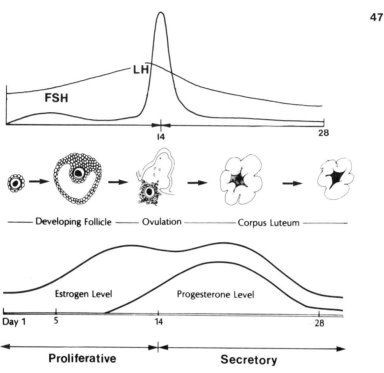

When the neurohormonal axis is functioning properly, there are pulsatile secretions of gonadotropin-releasing hormone from the hypothalamus (approximately every 90 min), which induce regular monthly cyclical secretions from the pituitary in the form of follicle-stimulating hormone (FSH) and luteinizing hormone (LH). The latter induce monthly ovulation from one of the ovaries.

FSH in the first half of the cycle (proliferative phase) induces the growth of several ovarian follicles; however, a dominant ovarian follicle emerges at approximately day 9, and the other follicles stop growing and then regress. The LH surge from the pituitary on day 14 or thereabouts causes ovulation from the single dominant ovarian follicle. During the second half of the cycle (secretory phase), the ovary continues to secrete estrogen, and the newly formed corpus luteum (which developed from the dominant ovarian follicle after ovulation) secretes increasing amounts of progesterone. These two ovarian hormones prepare the endometrium for possible implantation of a fertilized ovum during the secretory phase.

Normal Ovarian Morphology

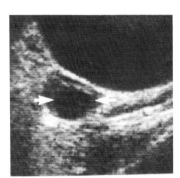

48. Sagittal scan of the right ovary on day 11. The mean diameter of the dominant ovarian follicle (*arrows*) is 1.3 cm.

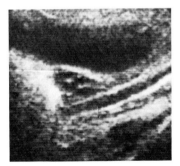

49. Sagittal scan of the same ovary on day 14. The mean diameter of the dominant ovarian follicle (*arrows*) is 2.0 cm.

50. Sagittal scan of the same ovary on day 15. The dominant follicle has ruptured, indicating that ovulation has occurred.

The most easily recognized morphological change during the menstrual cycle is the development and disappearance of the dominant ovarian follicle. The sequence shown in Figs. 48–50 is direct evidence that the reproductive neurohormonal axis is functioning normally.

Normal Ovarian Morphology

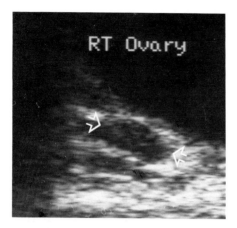

51. Sagittal scan of the right ovary in the 5-year-old girl: (*arrows*) upper and lower poles of the ovary; length, 1.1 cm; depth, 0.4 cm.

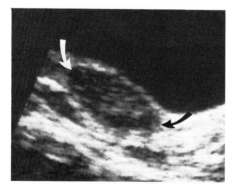

52. Sagittal scan of an ovary in a 20-year-old woman during the proliferative phase: (*arrows*) upper and lower poles of the ovary; length, 4.0 cm; depth, 1.9 cm.

In premenarchal girls, the ovary is small, ellipsoidal in shape, and often cyst-free; however, it is normal to see a few tiny follicular cysts in the premenarchal ovary. In postmenarchal women, the ovary is larger, ellipsoidal in shape, and often has small cystic structures (follicles) within it. In the proliferative phase, it is normal to visualize several tiny (2–6 mm diameter) follicles. Near midcycle, a dominant cyst (approximately 2-cm diameter) is usually visualized.

In the perimenopausal period, the ovary may contain follicular cysts, but when the menopause is established and the monthly hormonal cycling has ceased, the ovaries should be cyst-free.

Normal Ovarian Volume

$$\text{Volume} = 0.523 \times d_1 \times d_2 \times d_3$$

where d_1 is length; d_2 is depth; and d_3 is width.

	Ovarian volume (cc)	
Age	Mean	Range
Prepubertal		
(2–13 years)	0.1–1.0	0.1–6.5
Postmenarchal	9.0	5.7–18.0
Postmenopausal	3.5	0.8–7.0

The ovarian volume is calculated by using the simplified formula for a prolate ellipsoid. Up to 5 years of age, ovarian volume remains relatively stable; there is then steady growth in ovarian volume up to the time of menarche. During reproductive years, there is a wide range in normal ovarian volume. An ovary measuring up to approximately 18 cc may be considered normal if not accompanied by functional or morphological abnormality. For postmenopausal women, the following rule may be useful: A postmenopausal ovary that is two times the volume of the opposite ovary, or greater than 7 cc, should be further investigated.

Dominant Ovarian Follicle

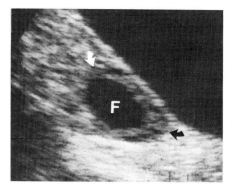

53. Sagittal scan of the ovary on the day before ovulation: (F) dominant follicle; (*arrows*) upper and lower poles of the ovary; maximum diameter of follicle, 2.5 cm; mean diameter, 2.0 cm. (*Note.* Normal ovarian tissue surrounds the follicle.)

In a normal 28-day cycle, a single dominant ovarian follicle may be observed to enlarge between day 9 and day 14. The *mean* diameter will increase during this time from 1.0 cm to 2.0 cm. When the *mean* follicular diameter reaches approximately 2 cm, ovulation is expected within the next 24 hr. Follow-up ultrasound can confirm ovulation by noting the disappearance of the dominant follicle *or* a large decrease in follicular size and alteration in shape. Following ovulation, there is usually a small amount of fluid in the cul-de-sac; however, fluid in the cul-de-sac is not a reliable sign of ovulation.

Corpus Luteum Cyst

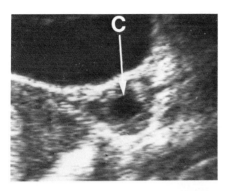

54. Transverse scan of pelvis: (C) corpus luteum cyst inside left ovary; diameter, 1.3 cm.

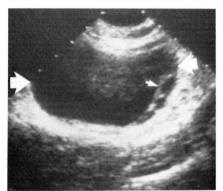

55. Sagittal scan through the left adnexa: (*large arrows*) 8-cm-diameter corpus luteum cyst (surgical proof); (*small arrow*) thin septations inside cyst.

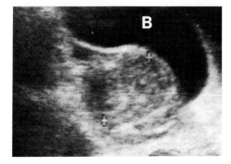

56. Sagittal scan through the left adnexa in another patient: (B) bladder; (+) a large hemorrhagic corpus luteum cyst. Ten days later, the left ovary was normal.

After ovulation, the empty cavity of the ruptured follicle is gradually filled by lutein cells, which become saturated with lipids. The corpus luteum may be difficult to identify sonographically. Not infrequently, however, it becomes cystic, and then it is easier to outline. The cyst is usually less than 2.5 cm in diameter, but we have seen much larger cysts (up to 8 cm in diameter) in otherwise normal women. By the onset of the next menses, the corpus luteum usually regresses and becomes atretic.

Hemorrhagic Ovarian Cyst

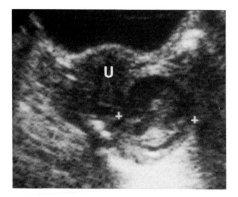

57. Transverse scan of the pelvis: (U) uterus; (+) complex mass in the left adnexa, representing a hemorrhagic corpus luteum cyst. This may be mistaken for an ectopic pregnancy with an embryo inside a gestational sac.

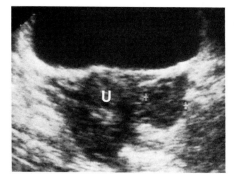

58. Transverse scan of the pelvis in the same patient 10 days later: (U) uterus; (+) normal left ovary.

A hemorrhagic cyst develops from a follicle or a corpus luteum by spontaneous rupture of blood vessels into the cystic cavity. The sonographic appearances are varied, ranging from a purely cystic lesion to a hyperechoic mass (simulating a solid lesion), a complex mass (partly hyperechoic and partly echo-free), or a septated cyst. To distinguish a hemorrhagic ovarian cyst from other surgical emergencies, we must often perform serial scans. In 7 to 10 days, a hemorrhagic cyst will usually change in internal characteristics and/or diminish in size.

Theca Lutein Cysts

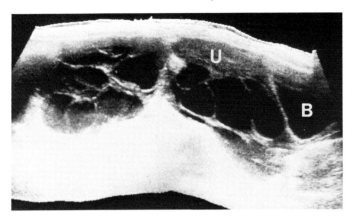

59. Sagittal scan of the abdomen and pelvis 2 days after evacuation of a hydatidiform mole from the uterus. Both ovaries are markedly enlarged by multiple theca lutein cysts. One ovary lies posterior to the uterus, and the other ovary lies cephalad to the uterus. Most of the observed septations are walls between adjacent cysts: (U) uterus; (B) bladder.

Theca lutein cysts may develop in conditions associated with increased levels of human chorionic gonadotropin (hCG), such as hydatidiform mole, choriocarcinoma, maternal–fetal Rh incompatibility (erythroblastosis fetalis), multiple pregnancies, and diabetes. There are a few reports of theca lutein cysts occurring in nonimmunologic fetal hydrops and in apparently normal pregnancies. Enlarged ovaries, containing multiple theca lutein cysts, may measure up to 20 cm in diameter. Large cysts may regress quite slowly after removal of the causative agent. Delayed regression is not a sign of persistent or recurrent trophoblastic disease.

Polycystic Ovaries

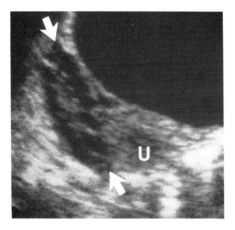

60. Transverse scan of the pelvis: (U) uterus; (*arrows*) right ovary containing multiple small cysts in the periphery of the ovary.

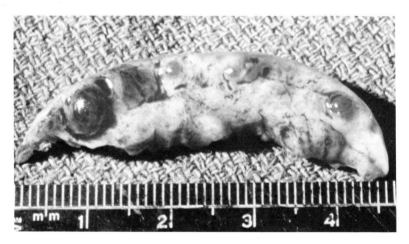

61. Wedge section from a "polycystic" ovary. Note the numerous small cysts in the periphery of the ovary.

Polycystic ovarian disease is better termed *chronic anovulation syndrome,* wherein dysfunctional hormonal cycles lead to chronic anovulation beginning at menarche. Clinical manifestations may also include hirsuitism, obesity, infertility, and oligomenorrhea. The morphology of polycystic ovaries is merely another sign of chronic anovulation.

Unfortunately, polycystic ovaries may be found in other conditions (e.g., adrenal tumors, birth control users), *and* the ovaries may be normal in chronic anovulation syndrome. However, in some patients with chronic anovulation, the typical morphology is present: large ovaries (>18 cc) and multiple (>10) peripheral cysts in each ovary (cysts range up to 6 or 7 mm in diameter).

Ovarian Hyperstimulation Syndrome (Drug-Induced)

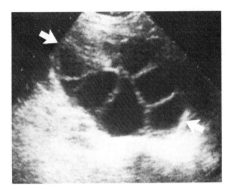

62. Sagittal scan of the right ovary: (*arrows*) right ovary measured 9.5 cm maximum diameter. It contains multiple large follicular cysts, which developed quickly during treatment with human menopausal gonadotropins. (*Note*. The echoes in one of the near-field cysts is due to reverberation artifact.)

Ovarian hyperstimulation syndrome (OHSS) is a relatively frequent complication in patients receiving drug therapy for infertility. The incidence ranges from 6% to 50%. The commonly used drugs are human menopausal gonadotropins (Pergonal) with subsequent human chorionic gonadotropins (hCGs) and clomiphene citrate (Clomid). The ovaries may become grossly enlarged and replaced by multiple *follicular* cysts of various sizes. In patients undergoing ovulation induction, ultrasound is used to document the number and size of the follicles. When three or more follicles greater than 1.5 cm are present, the chance of multiple pregnancies increases, and treatment may therefore be terminated at this point.

Pelvic Inflammatory Disease

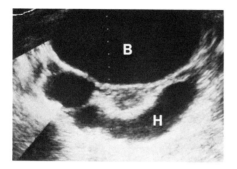

63. Hydrosalpinx; transverse scan of pelvis: (B) bladder; (H) tubular hydrosalpinx.

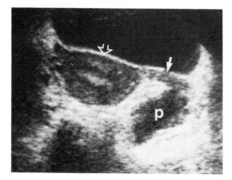

64. Pyosalpinx; transverse scan of pelvis: (*large arrow*) uterine fundus; (P) pyosalpinx involving distal end of the fallopian tube; (*small arrow*) proximal end of fallopian tube.

Pelvic inflammatory disease (PID) implies infection and inflammation involving the fallopian tubes and/or endometrium. Ultrasound can detect such complications of PID as hydrosalpinx, which is an accumulation of sterile fluid in a strictured tube; pyosalpinx, which is a dilated tube filled with pus; and tubo-ovarian abscess, where the abscess extends beyond the confines of the tube.

Pelvic Inflammatory Disease (*contd.*)

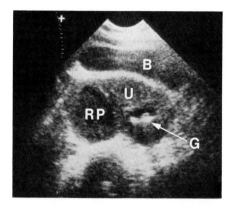

65. Pyosalpinx; transverse scan of pelvis: (B) bladder; (U) uterus; (RP) right pyosalpinx; (G) gas in left pyosalpinx.

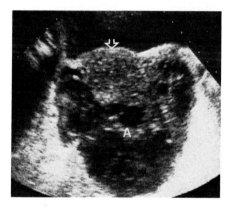

66. Tubo-ovarian abscess; transverse scan of pelvis: (*arrow*) uterine fundus; (A) large tubo-ovarian abscess in cul-de-sac.

The ultrasound appearance of a tubo-ovarian abscess is often nonspecific. It may be echo-free, complex, or mainly echogenic. If gas is present inside the collection, however, an abscess should be suspected.

Pelvic Endometriosis

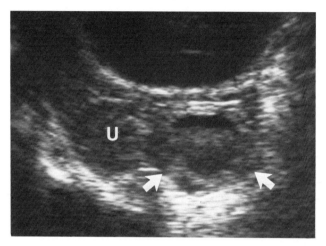

67. Transverse scan of pelvis: (U) uterine fundus; (*arrows*) large, thick-walled "chocolate cyst" of endometriosis in left adnexa. Dependent echogenic debris lies within the central liquified compartment.

This relatively common disorder is characterized by the presence of endometrial glands and/or stroma in locations outside the uterus. It affects 40% of infertile women. It is practically never seen in women over 50 years of age. The endometrial foci undergo cyclic menstrual changes with periodic bleeding, causing local blood collections (chocolate cysts or endometriomas) and fibroproliferative response in the involved organs. The role of ultrasound is limited to patients known to have endometriosis. Scans allow the detection of larger endometriomas and allow us to monitor their size over a period of time.

Ectopic Pregnancy

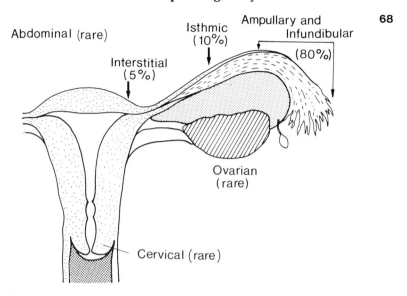

Ectopic pregnancy refers to implantation of the blastocyst in a location other than the endometrial cavity. The most common location is the fallopian tube (95% of cases), but implantation at other sites (although rare) is possible: the cervix, the ovary, and the abdominal cavity. The most common sites within the tube are the ampulla and infundibulum (fimbriated end); the most potentially dangerous location is the interstitial portion, where sudden, severe hemorrhage may occur. Although coexistent ectopic and intrauterine pregnancies do rarely occur, for practical purposes, the presence of an intrauterine gestation effectively rules out an ectopic pregnancy. The quoted incidences of coexistent ectopic and intrauterine pregnancies range from 1 in 6,800 to 1 in 30,000 pregnancies.

Ectopic Pregnancy: The Diagnostic Sonogram

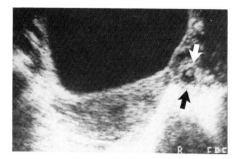

69. Transverse scan of the pelvis: (U) uterus, empty endometrial cavity; (*arrows*) gestational sac containing viable embryo. The crown–rump length suggests 8 to 9 weeks of gestation.

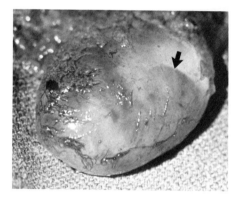

70. Intact gestational sac containing embryo. The implantation site was intact and embryo alive at surgery.

   The diagnostic finding is demonstration of an extrauterine adnexal gestational sac containing a viable fetus. Unfortunately, this diagnostic scan is rarely seen (less than 5%). Care must be taken not to confuse a blood clot in a hemorrhagic cyst with fetal parts.

Ectopic Pregnancy (*contd.*)

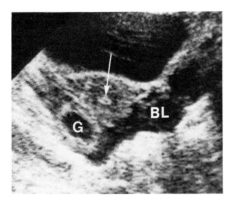

71. Transverse scan of the pelvis: (G) gestational sac surrounded by thick echogenic wall. The sac was in the fimbriated end of the fallopian tube; (BL) blood collection in the cul-de-sac: (*arrow*) empty endometrial cavity in the fundus of uterus.

In many patients the following features are seen on ultrasound:

1. an empty uterus;

2. an adnexal mass, which is variable in size and morphology depending on the age of the gestation and amount of local hemorrhage (the mass may be cystic, complex, or solid in appearance);

3. fluid in the peritoneal cavity.

With a positive pregnancy test and these findings, an ectopic pregnancy is highly probable.

Ectopic Pregnancy: Isthmic and Interstitial Ectopic Pregnancy

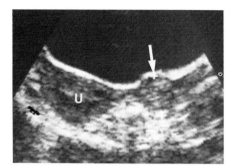

72. Isthmic ectopic pregnancy; transverse scan of the pelvis: (U) uterine fundus; (*arrow*) ectopic gestation (hemorrhagic) inside isthmic portion of the left fallopian tube. The left ovary was separate from this mass.

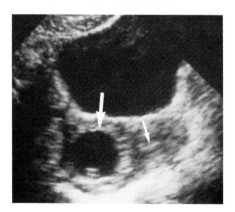

73. Interstitial ectopic pregnancy; transverse scan of the pelvis: (*long arrow*) gestational sac within the interstitial portion of the fallopian tube; (*short arrow*) uterus, empty endometrial cavity. A hysterectomy was performed because of severe pain and bleeding. The gestational sac was anembryonic (i.e., a "blighted ovum").

Diagnostic Pitfalls in Suspected Ectopic Pregnancy

Pregnancy test	False-positive ultrasound	False-negative ultrasound
Positive	Bicornuate uterus (fairly common) Early intrauterine pregnancy with corpus luteum cyst (common but rarely confusing)	Decidual cast mistaken for early intrauterine pregnancy (common) Viable extrauterine abdominal pregnancy (rare) Intrauterine and extrauterine pregnancy (rare) 1/30,000
Negative	Pelvic inflammatory disease Hemorrhagic ovarian cyst Endometriosis	False-negative pregnancy test (avoidable in most patients with β subunit of human chorionic gonadotropin

Modified and reproduced with permission from Hobbins JC, ed. *Diagnostic ultrasound in obstetrics.* New York: Churchill Livingstone, 1979:19.

Dermoid Tumor

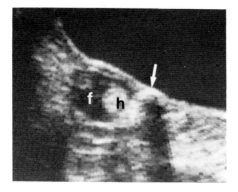

74. Sagittal scan demonstrating three different tissue types in a small (3 cm) dermoid tumor: (f) fluid-filled component; (h) hyperechoic portion without distal shadowing; (*arrow*) hyperechoic portion with distal shadowing. This was a tooth.

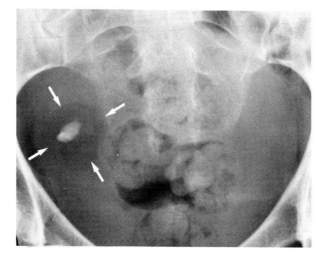

75. Radiograph of the pelvis of another patient: (*arrows*) fat density component of the dermoid tumor. (Note the well-defined tooth inside the fat component of the tumor.)

This is one of the few ovarian neoplasms that may show a diagnostic sonographic appearance. The signs are the following:

1. a hyperechoic focus within an adnexal mass with shadowing distal to the focus;

2. two or three different soft tissue elements within the mass, one of which is a collection of uniformly hyperechoic material (this usually represents sebacious material and/or hair).

In a few cases, we may see a highly reflective surface with shadowing obscuring everything posterior to it. This constitutes the "tip-of-the-iceberg" sign and is caused by highly reflective material in the near portion of the dermoid tumor.

Dermoid Tumor (*contd.*)

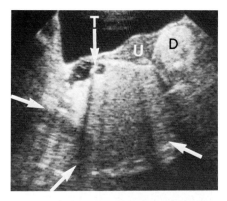

76. Bilateral dermoid tumors; transverse scan of the pelvis: (U) uterus; (D) left ovarian dermoid tumor; (*arrows*) right ovarian dermoid tumor; (T) tooth with distal acoustic shadowing. [*Note*. The echogenic internal material of the dermoids was sebaceous material. Also note the attenuation of sound in the right ovarian dermoid ("tip-of-the-iceberg" sign).]

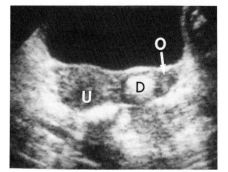

77. Transverse scan of the pelvis: (U) uterus; (D) small dermoid tumor (2 cm) in left ovary; (O) normal left ovarian tissue. (*Note*. The hyderdense material was sebaceous material.)

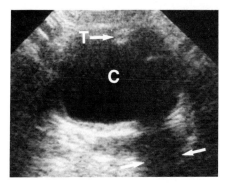

78. Cystic dermoid; sagittal scan of the pelvis: (C) cystic dermoid tumor; (*arrows*) acoustic shadow from a tooth in the anterior wall of the cystic dermoid; (T) tooth, which is difficult to visualize because of "noise" in the near field of the scan. (*Note*. Slightly thickened wall of cyst posteriorly.)

Cystic dermoid is a rare form of ovarian teratoma. In the majority of cases, one or more small solid nodules (dermoid plug) can be detected forming an acute angle with the wall of the cyst. These protuberances are outgrowths from the inner surface, containing hair and other tissues.

Cystadenoma and Cystadenocarcinoma

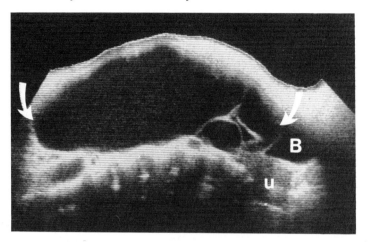

79. Mucinous cystadenoma; sagittal scan of the abdomen and pelvis: (B) bladder; (U) uterus; (*arrows*) huge mucinous cystadenoma with thin septations in caudal portion and low-level echoes (mucin) in cephalad portion.

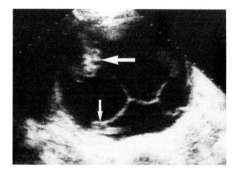

80. Serous cystadenocarcinoma; (*large arrow*) solid component arising from wall of tumor; (*small arrow*) thickening at the base of a septum.

Although not diagnostic, certain sonographic features are suggestive of these ovarian neoplasms:

1. The mass is predominantly cystic, with multiple fluid collections of different sizes separated by septae.

2. The mucinous cystadenoma may contain fine particulate material; it accounts for 16% to 30% of all benign ovarian neoplasms. Only 5% to 7% are bilateral, and only 5% to 10% become malignant.

3. The serous type is more often bilateral (30%–45%). There is a higher incidence of malignant transformation (30%–45%).

4. Solid masses lining the cystic walls (papillary growths) or thickened irregular septae should raise the suspicion of a cystadenocarcinoma.

Ovarian Carcinoma

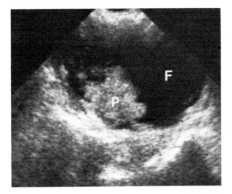

81. Papillary cystadenocarcinoma; scan of a large mass (8 cm diameter) in the pelvis, representing papillary cystadenocarcinoma: (F) fluid-filled component of tumor; (P) papillary solid component of tumor. (Note the lobulated or papillary contour of this component interfacing with the fluid component.)

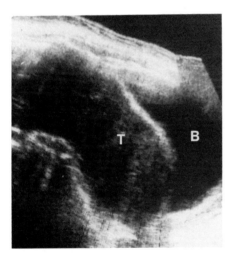

82. Solid ovarian carcinoma; sagittal scan of the pelvis: (B) bladder; (T) solid ovarian carcinoma filling the pelvis and extending into the lower abdomen.

Ultrasound may demonstrate evidence of advanced disease, such as large pelvic masses, peritoneal masses with ascites, and liver metastases. Note that ascites alone does not necessarily indicate peritoneal metastases in patients with known ovarian carcinoma. Ultrasound theoretically has the potential for early detection of ovarian carcinoma; however, there is no proof yet that ultrasound is an effective screening test for the early detection of ovarian malignancy.

Pelvic Varicosities

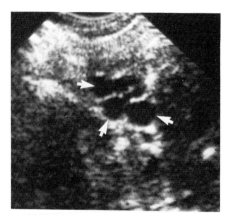

83. Transverse scan to the right of uterine fundus: (*arrows*) several serpiginous veins in the right adnexa.

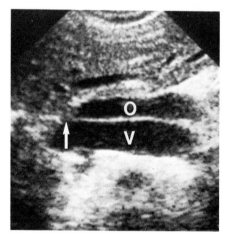

84. Sagittal scan in the right side of the abdomen in the same patient: (V) inferior vena cava; (O) right ovarian vein; (*arrow*) insertion site of right ovarian vein into inferior vena cava. The right ovarian vein is dilated, and it anastomosed with the varicosities in the right adnexa.

Dilated uterine and/or ovarian veins occur most commonly with or following pregnancy. Their tubular and serpiginous appearance as well as their location distinguish them from follicular cysts and hydroureters. Branches of the arcuate vein can occasionally be seen along the anterior or posterior uterine surface.

Pseudomass Due to Reverberation Artifact

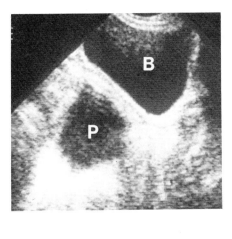

85. Sagittal scan of the pelvis: (B) bladder; (P) pseudomass.

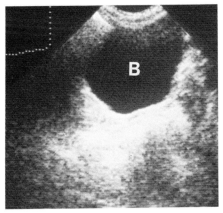

86. Sagittal scan of the same patient after decreasing the bladder volume slightly: (B) bladder. The pseudomass is no longer present.

In some pelvic sonograms, a pseudomass may appear posterior to the distended bladder due to reverberation of the sound beam within the bladder. The sound beam reflects from the posterior wall, then reflects from the anterior wall back toward the posterior wall, then reflects again from the posterior wall, and then is detected by the ultrasound probe. The resultant echo is printed at a depth twice the depth of the true posterior wall.

This artifact is suspected because the "mass" is too deep to be inside the pelvic cavity. The proof comes when the bladder volume is reduced, and the "mass" disappears because the shape of the bladder is altered.

Ectopic Pelvic Kidney

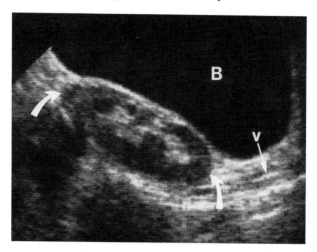

87. Sagittal scan of the pelvis: (B) bladder; (V) vaginal mucosa; (*arrows*) upper and lower poles of pelvic kidney.

Ectopic kidney usually lies anterior to the sacrum or ischium. It may be mistaken for an abnormal pelvic mass, although the morphology is usually that of a normal kidney. The diagnosis can be confirmed by an isotope renal scan if necessary.

Bowel

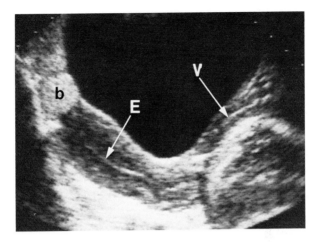

88. Sagittal scan of the pelvis: (V) vaginal mucosa; (E) endometrial cavity; (R) rectal contents; (b) bowel loop mimicking a solid mass. Peristalsis was observed, and a repeat scan 10 min later demonstrated no evidence of a mass.

Bowel loops in the pelvis are potential sources of confusion, especially in postsurgical patients or in patients with inflammatory bowel disease. Peristalsis when observed will help to exclude an inflammatory or neoplastic mass. Rescanning after introduction of fluid in the rectum can sometimes be useful.

In cases of suspected postoperative or posttraumatic abscess, however, computed tomographic (CT) scanning may be a better screening modality.

Rectus Sheath Hematoma

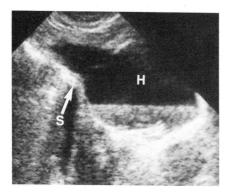

89. Sagittal scan of the pelvis: (H) large rectus sheath hematoma filling the pelvic cavity; (S) sacral promontory. *(Note.* Fluid-debris level in dependent portion of hematoma. Urinary bladder was empty and therefore not demonstrated.)

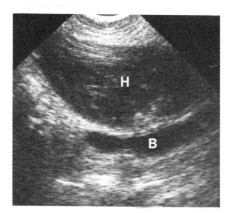

90. Sagittal scan of the pelvis in another patient: (H) hematoma of rectus sheath; (B) bladder displaced posteriorly.

Bleeding into the rectus sheath of the anterior abdominal wall may be due to trauma, surgery, blood dyscrasias (e.g., hemophilia), or anticoagulant therapy. Rectus sheath hematomas usually collect along the posterior aspect of the muscle belly and may be diagnosed via CT scans or small-parts ultrasound scanning of the anterior abdominal wall. Occasionally, however, the hematomas may become very large and impinge into the pelvis, simulating an intrapelvic mass. The two examples above demonstrate how hematomas of the anterior abdominal wall (posterior rectus sheath) may mimic an intrapelvic mass.

Appendiceal Abscess

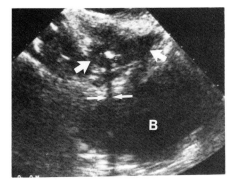

91. Oblique scan of the pelvis: (B) bladder; (+) fecalith; (*small arrows*) acoustic shadow posterior to fecalith; (*large arrows*) appendiceal abscess that was adherent to bladder wall at surgery.

An appendiceal abscess may simulate an adnexal mass. It is clinically difficult to distinguish from adnexal torsion or tubo-ovarian abscess. In certain cases, a diagnosis can be made sonographically by showing normal ovaries and by demonstrating a fecalith within the mass. This appearance may be confused with a dermoid tumor containing a tooth, but the clinical presentation often makes a distinction between these two diagnoses possible.

Chapter 6

EARLY PREGNANCY: EMBRYONIC PERIOD

Idealized Menstrual Cycle Before Pregnancy (28-Day Cycle)

Day	Event
0	Start of normal menstruation
14	Ovulation
14-16	Fertilization of ovum
21	Implantation in endometrium of uterine cavity
25-28	Sensitive pregnancy test becomes positive
35-42 (5-6 weeks)	Gestational sac detectable by ultrasound
35-42 (5-6 weeks)	Embryonic heart detectable with real-time ultrasound
42 (6 weeks)	Embryo and yolk sac detectable by ultrasound

The menstrual cycle lasts approximately 28 days. The start of the cycle is the first day of menstrual bleeding; ovulation occurs approximately 14 days before the beginning of the next cycle. In a 28-day cycle, ovulation occurs on day 14. In a longer cycle (e.g., 35 days), ovulation occurs later in the cycle (on day 21 of a 35-day cycle). The blastocyst actually implants before the next menstrual period is due, and sensitive pregnancy tests become positive 1 to 2 weeks before ultrasound can detect the gestational sac.

Conceptional age is the age of conceptus from fertilization. *Menstrual age* is the age of conceptus from the start of the last menstrual period. In clinical practice and in this book, we always mean *menstrual age* when we refer to weeks of gestation. The *embryonic period* encompasses up to 9 completed weeks of gestation.

Gestation: 5 Weeks (Schematic Diagram)

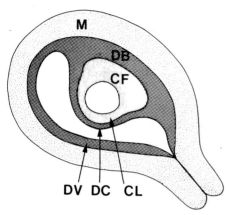

92. Sagittal diagram of a uterus containing a small gestation: (DB) decidua basalis; (DV) decidua vera; (DC) decidua capsularis; (CF) chorion frondosum; (CL) chorion laeve; (M) myometrium.

Decidua.   Transformed endometrial lining of the uterus during pregnancy.

Decidua basalis.   Thick decidua at the implantation site.

Decidua vera or *decidua perietalis.*   Decidua along the remainder of the uterine cavity beside the implantation site.

Decidua capsularis.   Thin decidua overlying the portion of the gastational sac facing the endometrial cavity.

Chorion.   Tissue lining the exterior of the gestational sac, derived from embryonic tissue. The purpose of the chorion is to "invade" the decidua to establish nutrition for the embryo.

Chorion frondosum.   Chorion at the implantation site.

Chorion laeve.   The thin chorion covering the portion of the gestational sac facing the endometrial cavity.

Gestation: 5 Weeks

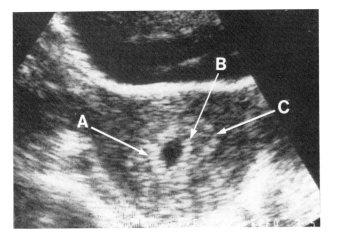

93. Axial scan of the uterus containing a small gestational sac: (A) decidua basalis plus chorion frondosum; (B) decidua capsularis plus chorion laeve; (C) decidua vera.

At the menstrual age of approximately 5 weeks, a gestational sac may be seen before an embryo or yolk sac is visible. To distinguish this from any other fluid collection, we must identify the two concentric rings that comprise the decidua chorionic ring (DCR) sign. The inner ring is the decidua capsularis plus the chorion laeve. The outer ring is the decidua vera. At the implantation site, the hyperechoic rim is thicker, and it comprises the decidua basalis and chorion frondosum.

Gestation: 5 to 7 Weeks

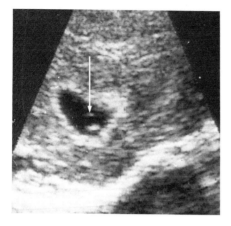

94. Sonogram at 5½ weeks of gestation: (*arrow*) secondary fetal yolk sac inside gestational sac.

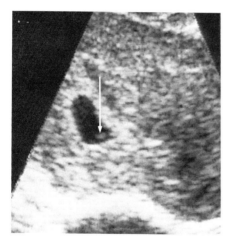

95. Sonogram at 6 weeks of gestation. (*arrow*) embryo. Cardiac activity was observed during real-time scan.

Between 5 and 6 weeks of gestation, the secondary fetal yolk sac becomes visible, whereas the embryo may not be visible. However, the embryonic heart activity may still be appreciated in magnified views by closely inspecting the area adjacent to the yolk sac. This will confirm a viable embryo despite lack of visualization of the embryo per se. At 6 weeks (menstrual age), the embryo becomes detectable with current ultrasound equipment. The secondary fetal yolk sac can also be seen and is usually 5 to 6 mm in diameter.

Gestation: 7 to 9 Weeks

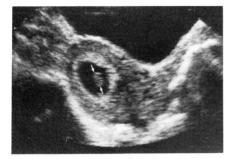

96. Sagittal scan of the uterus: (*arrows*) demarcation of the crown–rump length, which measures 1.0 cm, consistent with 7 weeks of gestation.

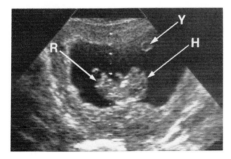

97. Transverse scan of the uterus demonstrating an embryo in supine position. The crown–rump length is 2.8 cm, consistent with 9½ weeks of gestation: (R) bottom of rump; (H) top of head; (Y) yolk sac.

Between 7 and 9 weeks of gestation, the embryonic head and rump become distinguishable. The distance from the top of the head to the bottom of the rump is called the crown–rump length (CRL), and it can predict the gestational age (GA) within ±4 days. The first scan demonstrates an embryo with a CRL of 1.0 cm, which predicts a gestational age of 7 weeks (±4 days). The second scan demonstrates an embryo with a CRL of 2.8 cm, which predicts a gestational age of 9 weeks and 3 days (±4 days).

As a rough rule of thumb, the following formula can be used to calculate GA from CRL:

$$GA \text{ (weeks)} = CRL \text{ (cm)} + 6.5$$

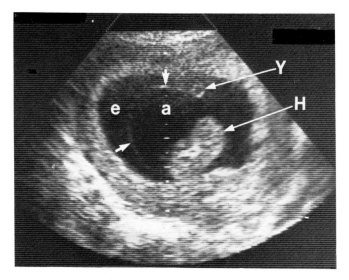

98. (a) Amniotic fluid; (e) extraembryonic celomic fluid; (Y) yolk sac; (H) head of embryo; (*arrows*) amniotic membrane.

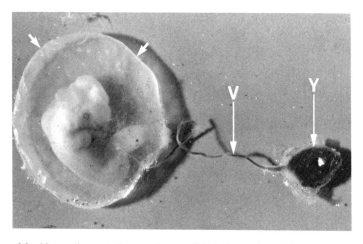

99. (*Arrows*) amniotic membrane; (V) vitelline duct; (Y) yolk sac.

A menstrual age of 10 weeks marks the end of the embryonic period. The amniotic membrane is a thin membrane that is still separate from the chorionic membrane. The crown–rump length is still the most accurate measurement in predicting menstrual age. The biparietal diameter becomes useful for dating at approximately 12 weeks of gestation.

Twins

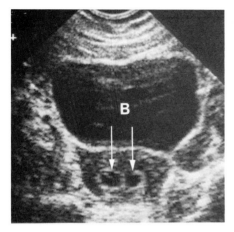

100. Transverse scan of the uterine fundus with the transducer placed on the midline of the patient: (B) urinary bladder; (*arrows*) apparently two separate gestational sacs inside the uterus. Two separate fetal heart beats were seen.

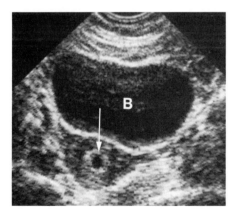

101. Transverse scan of the same uterus with the transducer placed beside the midline of the patient: (B) urinary bladder; (*arrow*) only one gestational sac is actually inside uterus. (Note the true width of the uterus in this image compared to the scan above.)

Twins may be diagnosed from 6 weeks of gestation and beyond. Although one twin may succumb at an early stage, most viable twins diagnosed even as early as 6 weeks will survive beyond the embryonic period. Care must be taken to avoid a false diagnosis of twins:

1. A collection of fluid (blood) may be present beside the gestational sac.
2. In a transverse scan taken in the midline, a split image may give the appearance of twins (split-image artifact shown above).

Blighted Ovum

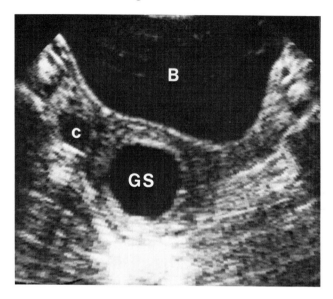

102. Transverse scan of the uterine fundus containing a large gestational sac but no evidence of an embryo: (B) urinary bladder; (C) cyst in right ovary (probably a corpus luteum cyst of pregnancy); (GS) gestational sac. The mean diameter of the gestational sac was 3.2 cm.

A better term for blighted ovum is *anembryonic gestation*. The very early embryo succumbs for some reason (at 4–5 weeks). An apparently empty gestational sac is demonstrated, often larger than expected for a normal sac without a visible embryo. If the mean diameter of the gestational sac is greater than 2.5 cm *and* an embryo is not visible, then the diagnosis of a blighted ovum can be made with confidence.

Where the diagnosis is not certain, a repeat scan should be performed in approximately 10 days. If a normal pregnancy is present, the embryo will become visible at the next scan. If a blighted ovum is present, no embryo will be seen at the next scan.

Bleeding in Early Pregnancy

Time[a]	Explanation	Ultrasound
3-4 Weeks	Implantation bleeding	Perhaps some fluid in endometrial cavity. Gestational sac *not* visible at this stage
5-20 Weeks	Missed abortion	Visible embryo. No embryonic activity. Perhaps disorganization of gestational sac and embryo
5-20 Weeks	Incomplete abortion	Some retained products of conception. Usually products of conception are nonspecific disorganized material
10-20 Weeks	Early subchorionic hematoma; placental abruption	A fairly common occurrence. Usually echo-poor crescentic fluid collection beside gestational sac. Embryo usually alive
5-20 Weeks	Other	Ectopic pregnancy Hydatidiform mole Cervical lesions (not usually detected with ultrasound)

[a]Time passed since the beginning of the last normal menstrual period.

Missed Abortion

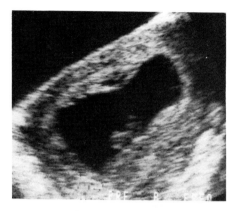

103. Transverse scan of the uterine fundus, which contains a relatively small embryo with no sign of embryonic life. There was no embryonic growth in the previous three weeks.

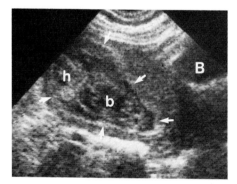

104. Sagittal scan of uterus: (B) urinary bladder; (*arrows*) endometrial lining of uterus. A nonviable fetus lies inside the uterine cavity. The fetal head and body are difficult to recognize if death has occurred many days earlier: (h) fetal head; (b) fetal body.

A missed abortion occurs when there is death of the embryo or fetus (less than 20 weeks of gestation), but the entire gestation remains *in utero.* Clinically, there may be vaginal bleeding, but no tissue has passed per vaginum. In recent death, the embryo and sac may appear to be normal except for lack of embryonic or fetal activity. In long-standing cases, the embryo and gestational sac become smaller and more disorganized.

Incomplete Abortion

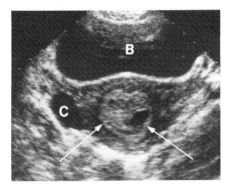

105. Transverse scan of uterine fundus: (B) urinary bladder; (C) corpus luteum cyst of pregnancy; (*arrows*) partly hyperechoic and partly anechoic material inside uterine cavity. No recognizable fetal parts were present.

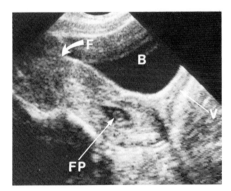

106. Sagittal scan of the uterus: (B) urinary bladder; (F) fundus of uterus; (FP) fetal part in lower uterine segment; (V) vagina. (*Note.* Remainder of products of conception passed spontaneously 1 hr after the ultrasound scan.)

Incomplete abortion occurs when the embryo or fetus has died, and some products of conception have been passed per vaginum. In many cases, the retained products within the uterus appear nonspecific and disorganized. The material may represent chorionic tissue, embryonic tissue, and/or decidual tissue. Given the ultrasound images alone, it is usually not possible to make this diagnosis with certainty.

Chapter 7

THE PLACENTA

Normal Placenta: First Trimester (10 Weeks)

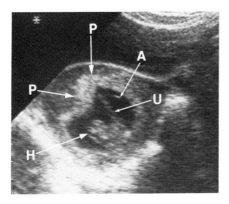

107. Transverse scan of uterine fundus: (H) head of embryo; (P) placenta; (A) amniotic membrane; (U) umbilical cord.

As early as 8 or 9 weeks of gestation, the placenta may be identified sonographically as a uniformly hyperechoic band of tissue. The tissue is made up of the decidua basalis and chorion frondosum. Although the placenta often seems close to the cervix, the diagnosis of placenta previa cannot be made with confidence at this early stage. What appears to be a placenta previa in the first trimester often is clearly not a placenta previa on reexamination in the third trimester.

Normal Placenta: Third Trimester (30 Weeks)

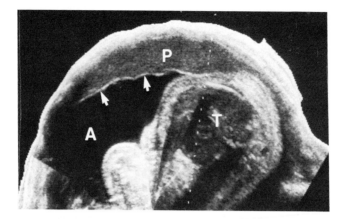

108. Transverse static scan of the pregnant uterus: (*arrows*) chorionic plate of the placenta; (A) amniotic fluid; (P) placenta; (T) thorax of fetus.

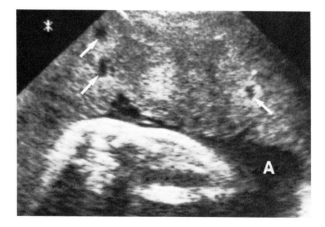

109. Scan through another placenta in third trimester: (A) amniotic fluid; (*arrows*) hypoechoic foci ("holes") in placenta, surrounded by hyperechoic material. These foci are seen in some normally maturing placentas in third trimester.

In the second and third trimesters, most placentas maintain their uniform pattern of echogenicity. The chorionic plate forms the fetal surface of the placenta, and it usually appears as a well-defined hyperechoic line. The underlying myometrium can be distinguished from the placenta, and the position of the placenta can be established with respect to the cervix.

It is possible to calculate placental volumes, but this practice is not very useful. A more practical gauge of placental size is the thickness determined near its midportion. A placental thickness greater than 5 cm in the third trimester is indicative of an abnormally large placenta.

Venous Structures

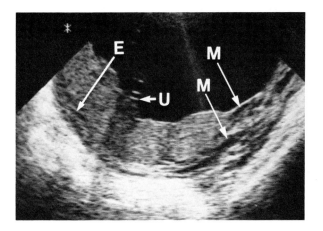

110. (E) Endometrial veins at base of placenta; (U) umbilical vein at insertion site into placenta; (M) marginal veins at edge of placenta.

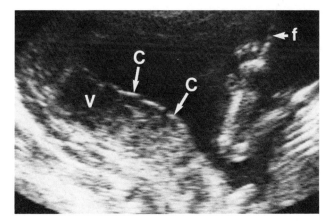

111. (V) Venous complex at edge of placenta; (C) chorionic plate of placenta; (f) second finger of fetal hand.

Veins can be seen at the base of the placenta (endometrial veins), at the margins of the placenta, within placental tissue, and beneath the chorionic plate of the placenta. On static images these appear as echo-free or hypoechoic spaces, and they can be confused with abnormal collections of fluid. However, on real-time examination with increased gain settings, we can usually demonstrate the slow swirling motion of the blood flow within them and thus confirm that they are normal venous structures.

Note that intravascular blood is slightly more echogenic than urine or amniotic fluid. By increasing the total gain of the ultrasound machine, this difference will become apparent.

Venous Structures (*contd.*)

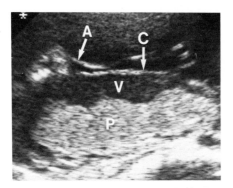

112. (A) Amniotic membrane; (C) chorionic plate; (P) placental tissue; (V) venous lake beneath chorionic plate. Slow swirling motion was observed within venous lake during real-time scanning.

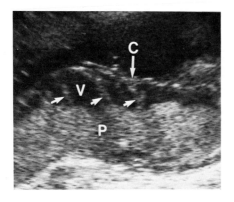

113. (C) Chorionic plate; (V) venous lakes beneath chorionic plate; (*arrows*) septae dividing venous lake into compartments; (P) placental tissue.

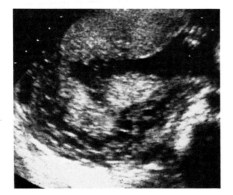

114. Prominent (but normal) endometrial veins are present at the base of the placenta.

Calcifications

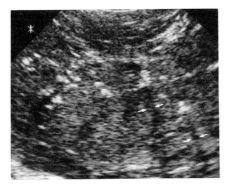

115. An oblique scan through placental tissue at 37 weeks of gestation. Multiple hyperechoic (*white*) foci represent placental calcifications; (*arrows*) faint acoustic shadowing posterior to some calcifications.

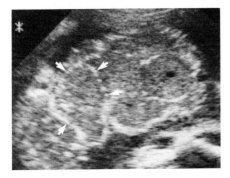

116. Sonogram in another patient at 30 weeks of gestation: (*arrows*) linear calcifications outlining a placental lobule. This represents a grade 3 placenta.

Placental calcification is uncommon before the third trimester; however, from 32 weeks until full term, the incidence of calcification in normal placentas increases to more than 50%. Calcifications may be extensive and involve the basal plate, the interlobular septae, and the subchorionic area. It is possible to grade placentas (grades 0, 1, 2, 3) depending on the degree of calcification. Extensive calcification (grade 3) was thought to be an excellent sign of fetal pulmonary maturity; however, this is not strictly true. Pulmonary immaturity may be present with a grade 3 placenta. Pulmonary maturity appears to be independently related to gestational age but *not* independently related to the degree of placental calcification.

The curvilinear calcifications occur in septae that separate placental lobes. They *do not* outline cotyledons, which are functional placental units that are not recognizable morphologically.

Succenturiate Lobe

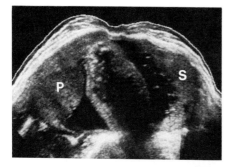

117. Transverse sonogram of uterus: (P) main portion of placenta implanted on the right uterine wall; (S) succenturiate lobe of placenta implanted on left uterine wall.

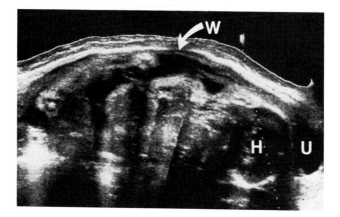

118. Sagittal midline sonogram. There is no evidence of placental tissue in the midline connecting the two masses of placental tissue: (W) wall of uterus; (H) head of fetus; (U) urinary bladder.

This accessory lobe appears physically separate from the main placenta. It is uncommon (approximately 1% or 2% of pregnancies), but its identification is important for two main reasons: (a) to rule out placental tissue overlying the internal cervical os; and (b) to avoid retained placental tissue at delivery.

The two masses of placental tissue are connected by vessels coursing beneath the common chorionic plate. Occasionally these connecting vessels may overlie the cervical os (vasa previa), and this can lead to severe bleeding during labor and delivery.

Subchorionic Fibrin Deposition

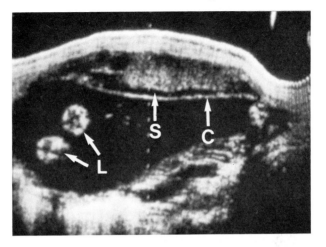

119. (L) Limbs of fetus in cross section; (C) chorionic plate; (S) subchorionic space containing few or no echoes. In the absence of demonstrable blood flow within this space, this could be subchorionic fibrin deposition or a hematoma.

An echo-free (or hypoechoic) space beneath the chorionic plate of the placenta may represent a venous lake, a subchorionic hematoma, or a deposit of fibrin tissue. Flow within the collection allows a diagnosis of a venous lake (which has no clinical significance), but the distinction between a hematoma and a fibrin deposit is very difficult. The fibrin deposit is probably the end result of a previous subchorionic thrombosis within a venous space. Intraplacental fibrin deposition and intraplacental hematomas rarely occur, and they appear as echo-free or echo-poor areas without evidence of venous flow within them.

Complete Hydatidiform Mole

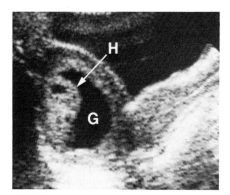

120. Sagittal sonogram of uterus: (H) hydatidiform mole impinging into gestational sac; (G) gestational sac; anechoic fluid fills the majority of endometrial cavity.

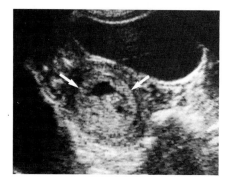

121. Oblique sonogram of the uterus in another patient: (*arrows*) molar tissue filling most of endometrial cavity. Two or three small anechoic spaces represent molar vesicles or, possibly, collections of blood.

The ultrasound of an early hydatidiform mole may be indistinguishable from a missed or incomplete abortion. The material inside the endometrial cavity may be mainly hyperechoic or mainly echo-free; however, as in all patients with a complete mole, the serum β-human chorionic gonadotropin level should be markedly elevated.

Complete Hydantidiform Mole (*contd.*)

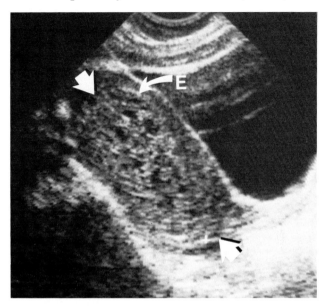

122. Sagittal sonogram of the uterus: (E) endometrial lining in anterior fundus; (*arrows*) demarcates the extent of molar tissue filling and distending the endometrial cavity. Multiple anechoic (*black*) areas represent vesicles or, possibly, hematomas.

Complete or classical hydatidiform mole represents complete replacement of placental tissue with molar tissue. The patient often presents with abnormal bleeding in the first trimester, and the uterus may be large, normal, or small-for-dates. Ultrasound often demonstrates hyperechoic material interspersed with tiny fluid-filled vesicles and, possibly, hematomas inside the uterine cavity. In approximately 50% of patients, septated theca lutein cysts of the ovary may also be demonstrated. A fetus or embryo is not present in a complete mole, with one exception: in a twin gestation where one twin is normal and the other pregnancy is replaced by a complete hydatidiform mole.

Recurrent or Invasive Hydatidiform Mole

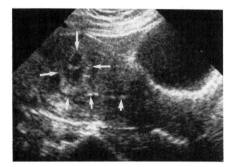

123. Sagittal sonogram of the uterus: (*long arrows*) abnormal mass (partly hyperechoic and partly hypoechoic) adjacent to endometrial lining; (*short arrows*) endometrium.

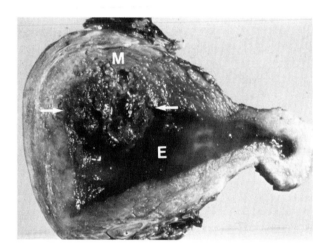

124. Pathological specimen of the uterus: (*arrows*) molar tissue invading myometrium; (M) myometrium; (E) endometrial cavity.

After evacuation of a complete mole, the best way to assess for possible local recurrence or distant metastases is to evaluate serial serum β-human chorionic gonadotropin (hCG) levels. After evacuation, the serum β-hCG levels should decrease exponentially with time in those free of disease. At ultrasound, recurrent or invasive mole may present as a focus of hyperechoic material containing tiny cysts inside the endometrial cavity or within the myometrium. Scans of the liver should also be made to rule out liver metastases.

Partial Hydatidiform Mole

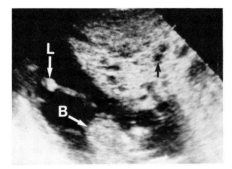

125. Scan through placenta demonstrates multiple "cystic" lesions within placental tissue: (L) limb of fetus; (B) body of fetus; (*arrow*) one of the multiple cysts within the placenta. Chromosome analysis later demonstrated fetal triploidy (i.e., 3 sets of chromosomes instead of the normal 2 sets of chromosomes).

Molar tissue replacing a part of the placenta may occur, and it is often associated with fetal triploidy (three complete sets of chromosomes instead of two). Ultrasound demonstrates a placenta that is partly normal and partly replaced by molar tissue. The coexistent fetus can be identified.

In some patients with a missed abortion or incomplete abortion, small areas of cystic degeneration may be seen in the retained placenta. This cystic degeneration is thought to be unrelated to the complete hydatidiform mole or the partial hydatidiform mole.

In a partial mole, there is low probability of metastases, invasion, or recurrence after the delivery; however, because rare cases of recurrence have been published, we should monitor serum β-human chorionic gonadotropin levels in these patients.

Chorioangioma

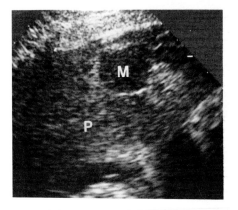

126. (M) Mass representing chorioangioma within base of placental tissue; (P) placental tissue.

Chorioangiomas are benign tumors that arise in the placenta from chorionic and vascular tissue, and they are quite common at full term. However, because many are small and because their echogenicity is similar to normal placentas, they are infrequently recognized on ultrasound scans. Larger tumors will be visualized and on rare occasions may cause significant vascular shunts, which could lead to fetal hydrops and polyhydramnios.

Large Placenta

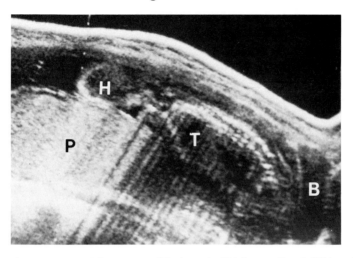

127. Sagittal scan of the uterus: (P) placenta (thickness, 6 cm); (H) head of fetus; (T) thorax of fetus; (B) maternal bladder.

The normal placenta is usually less than 5 cm thick across the central portion during the third trimester. Causes of a thickened or enlarged placenta include Rh isoimmunization, maternal diabetes, maternal anemia, and congenital infections.

In Rh disease, other changes, such as polyhydramnios and fetal hydrops, may be present at the same time. With a large placenta associated with maternal diabetes, there may also be polyhydramnios and increased fetal weight, with excess subcutaneous fetal fat visible.

Early Placenta Previa

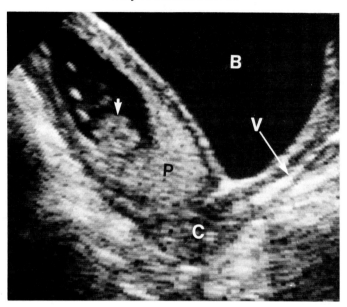

128. Sagittal scan of the uterus at 15 weeks of gestation, demonstrating a central placenta previa: (arrow) fetal abdomen; (P) placenta; (C) cervix; (V) vagina; (B) bladder. (Note. At full term, the internal cervical os was covered by placental tissue.)

Apparent early placenta previas (less than 20 weeks of gestation) often become clear of the cervix in the third trimester. This is usually true where the margin of the placenta appears to be at the internal os. This apparent placental migration away from the cervix is probably related to the development and elongation of the lower uterine segment in later pregnancy; however, when there is definite evidence of placental tissue overlying the internal cervical os after 20 weeks of gestation, this positioning often persists until delivery and represents a clinically significant placenta previa. Vaginal delivery is contraindicated.

Occasionally, a central placenta previa appears to be present (i.e., the central portion of the placenta appears to overlie the internal cervical os) at less than 20 weeks. It is quite possible that this will persist as a placenta previa at full term.

Marginal Placenta Previa

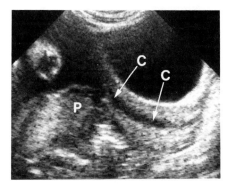

129. Sagittal scan of the lower uterine segment and cervix. Margin of placenta lies very close to internal cervical os but does not cover the os (marginal placenta previa): (P) placenta; (C) cervical canal.

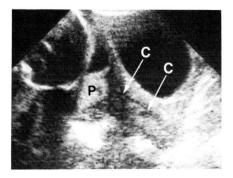

130. Sagittal scan of lower uterine segment and cervix. Margin of placenta covers internal os of cervix (complete placenta previa): (P) placenta; (C) cervical canal.

In the third trimester, the margin of the placenta may lie either at the apparent position of the internal cervical os or very close to it. It is important to alter the bladder volume to optimize visualization of the cervix and placenta. An overdistended bladder may compress the anterior and posterior lower uterine segments together and give the false appearance of a placenta previa.

Complete placenta previa. Entire internal cervical os is covered by placental tissue.

Central placenta previa. A type of complete previa where the central part of the placenta covers the internal os.

Partial placenta previa. Part of the internal os is covered by placental tissue. This condition is established by digital examination but cannot be diagnosed by ultrasound.

Marginal placenta previa. A term derived from digital examination wherein the internal os is free of placenta, but the placental margin is within reach of the examiner's finger (i.e., the placental margin is within approximately 3 cm of the edge of the internal os).

Subchorionic Hematoma and Placental Abruption: 9 to 20 Weeks

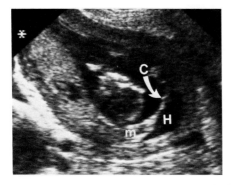

131. (m) Margin of placenta; (C) chorionic membrane; (H) hematoma.

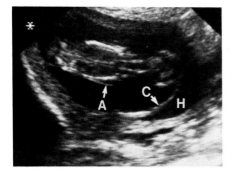

132. (A) Amniotic membrane; (C) chorionic membrane; (H) hematoma.

A subchorionic hematoma is a fairly common occurrence between 9 and 20 weeks of gestation. It usually occurs spontaneously in an otherwise normal pregnancy without evidence of a placenta previa. In small hematomas (calculated volume less than 60 cc), the prognosis is good (that is, high probability of progressing to full term). Follow-up scans usually demonstrate gradual (2 or more weeks) resorption of the hematoma and normal growth of the fetus. In approximately 60% of patients with a subchorionic hematoma, the margin of placenta is observed to be separated from the underlying uterine wall.

Subchorionic Hematoma and Placental Abruption:
20 to 40 Weeks

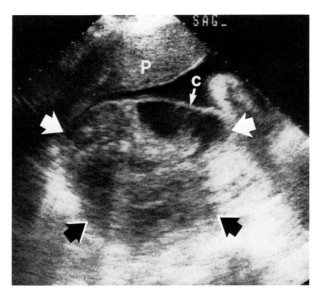

133. (P) Placenta; (C) chorionic membrane; (*arrows*) large subchorionic hematoma. The placental implantation appeared intact.

In clinical obstetric practice, placental abruption in later pregnancy is not uncommon, but ultrasound abnormalities are usually not seen in these cases. However, in patients with positive sonograms, we may observe a subchorionic hematoma separate from the placenta, separation of the placental margin, a retroplacental hematoma, or even an intraplacental extension of the hematoma. The hematoma may be almost echo-free, or it may evolve to contain echoes and then be confused with myometrial or placental tissue.

Chapter 8

THE MEMBRANES, AMNIOTIC FLUID, AND UMBILICAL CORD

Chorioamniotic Separation

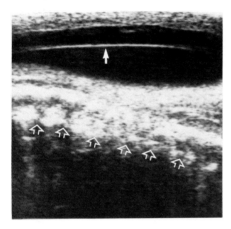

134. Sagittal scan of the uterus, 39 weeks of gestation: (*arrow*) amniotic membrane; (*open arrows*) fetal spine.

The amniotic membrane delineates the margins of the amniotic cavity surrounding the fetus. The chorionic membrane delineates the margins of the chorionic cavity that surrounds the amniotic cavity. The amniotic cavity grows more rapidly than the chorionic cavity, resulting in obliteration of the chorionic cavity at approximately 16 weeks of menstrual age. Therefore, visualization of a thin, mobile amniotic membrane up to this gestation is normal and is referred to as chorioamniotic separation (CAS).

CAS may be seen in later pregnancy. It is usually due to a tear in the amnion, resulting in leaking of fluid with separation of the amniotic and chorionic membranes. The most common cause is trauma, usually of iatrogenic nature. It is usually not of clinical significance.

Amniotic Band Syndrome

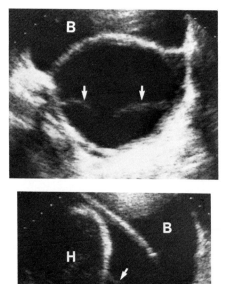

135. Transverse scan of the uterus: (B) bladder; (*arrows*) amniotic band.

136. Sagittal scan of the uterus: (B) bladder; (H) fetal head; (*arrows*) amniotic band.

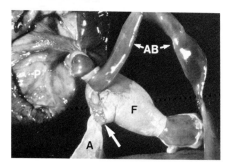

137. Pathological specimen of another fetus with amniotic band syndrome demonstrating marked constriction of fetal arm due to arm entrapment: (P) placenta; (AB) amniotic band; (*arrow*) band around fetal arm; (A) arm; (F) forearm.

Amniotic band syndrome represents part of the amniotic membrane disruption complex. When amniotic membrane disruption occurs, adhesions develop between the amniotic and chorionic membranes. If a fetal part passes through the defect in the amnion, adhesions may develop between the chorionic membrane and the fetal part. Constriction of the fetal part by the adhesion can cause a spectrum of abnormalities varying from simple edema to hypoplasia to amputation. The fetal entrapment represents the amniotic band syndrome. If the fetus is free and mobile, the membrane or band is probably benign. We may see a short umbilical cord secondary to prolonged decreased fetal movement.

Membranes in Multiple Gestation

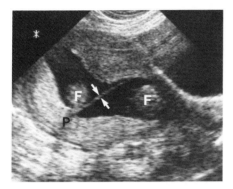

138. Sagittal scan of uterus, diamniotic–monochorionic twins: (*arrows*) membrane separating the two amniotic cavities; (P) placenta.

A membrane should be carefully sought in multiple gestation. It may be difficult to demonstrate in late pregnancy. Monoamniotic–monochorionic twins (a single amniotic sac and a single placenta) occur in 1% to 5% of all twin gestations. When a membrane is absent between the fetuses, there is a high risk of cord entanglement, which could have catastrophic results, with a 50% to 70% mortality rate.

Amniotic Fluid: Normal

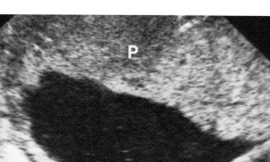

139. Transverse scan of the uterus: (P) placenta. Note the particulate matter within the amniotic fluid.

There is an absolute increase in volume of amniotic fluid up to approximately 38 weeks of menstrual age. There is a relative decrease in volume of amniotic fluid during the third trimester. Particulate matter consisting of vernix and/or cellular debris is normally seen in the second half of pregnancy. It cannot be differentiated from meconium. A normal volume of amniotic fluid is recognized by exclusion of hydramnios or oligohydramnios.

Amniotic Fluid Volume

140. *Hydramnios (or polyhydramnios):* (*arrows*) excessive fluid separates the uterine wall from the fetal body; (F) fetal chest.

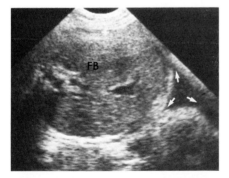

141. *Normal amniotic fluid volume.* Transverse scan of the fetal abdomen: (*arrows*) pocket of amniotic fluid that measured 2.5 cm in greatest diameter; (FB) fetal body. Larger pockets were also present.

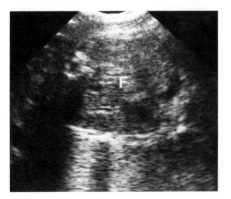

142. *Oligohydramnios.* Transverse scan of the fetal abdomen: (F) fetal abdomen. There is a marked paucity of fluid around the fetus.

Hydramnios

Hydramnios (polyhydramnios) is an excessive volume of amniotic fluid during the third trimester. It occurs in approximately 0.7% of all deliveries. Amniotic fluid volume is very difficult to quantitate. The following are subjective ultrasound features of hydramnios:

1. The anterior uterine wall is displaced away from the fetal body by amniotic fluid. This is the most reliable sign.
2. The fetal limbs are easily seen due to excessive fluid.
3. The umbilical cord is easily seen.

Conditions Associated with Hydramnios

Associated conditions	Approximate percentage
Idiopathic	33
Maternal	
Diabetes mellitus (most common single associated condition, 20%)	
Preeclampsia	40
Rh isoimmunization	
Fetal	
CNS disorders form the majority of the fetal group	
Anencephaly (80% of CNS group)	
Neural tube defects	
Hydrocephalus	20
Gastrointestinal disorders form most of the remainder	
Esophageal obstruction without tracheo-esophageal fistula	
Duodenal obstruction	
Proximal small bowel obstruction	
Other	
Fetal–fetal transfusion syndrome in monozygotic twins (uncommon)	7
Many rare associated conditions	

Oligohydramnios

Oligohydramnios means that too little amniotic fluid is present. Oligohydramnios occurs in approximately 4% of all pregnancies. Ultrasound features of oligohydramnios are the following:

1. The largest pocket of amniotic fluid measures less than 2 cm in greatest diameter.
2. Crowding of fetal parts in the second trimester.
3. The uterine wall is closely applied to the fetus without apparent intervening fluid in the second or early third trimester.

(There is a considerable subjective element to items 2 and 3.)

Accurate estimation of percentage association with other conditions is not available; however, the following will serve as a rough guideline:

1. Intrauterine growth retardation (IUGR) occurs when a fetus is small for gestational age. A newborn baby that is less than the tenth percentile weight for gestational age has mild IUGR. Using this definition, IUGR occurs in 8% to 10% of all pregnancies. It can be suspected *in utero* when the estimated fetal weight is less than the tenth percentile for gestational age or when oligohydramnios is present. Excluding patients with premature rupture of membranes, approximately 83% of patients with oligohydramnios will have IUGR; however, only approximately 16% of patients with IUGR fetuses will have oligohydramnios. IUGR is more common in younger, nulliparous patients who are smokers and are hypertensive. Fetal weight should be calculated whenever oligohydramnios is present.
2. Maternal causes are the next most common group. Premature rupture of membranes can cause severe oligohydramnios or anhydramnios. Postmaturity and chronic leak of amniotic fluid can also cause oligohydramnios.
3. Fetal causes are usually related to urinary tract abnormalities. Bilateral renal aplasia (Potter's syndrome) will cause anhydramnios before 20 weeks of gestation. Bilateral multicystic dysplastic kidney, infantile polycystic kidney disease, and urethral obstruction are the other uncommon but important anomalies causing this condition.

The Umbilical Cord: Three-Vessel Cord

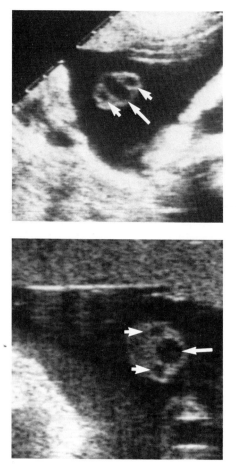

143 and 144. Normal three-vessel cord; transverse scan of umbilical cord: (*large arrow*) vein; (*small arrows*) arteries.

Three-Vessel Cord

The normal umbilical cord is 1 to 2 cm in diameter in the third trimester. It contains one large vein and two smaller arteries surrounded by Wharton's jelly, which is a myxomatous connective tissue. Wharton's jelly is deposited mainly during the sixth to eighth months of pregnancy and decreases thereafter. The cord is covered by the amnion.

The Umbilical Cord: Two-Vessel Cord

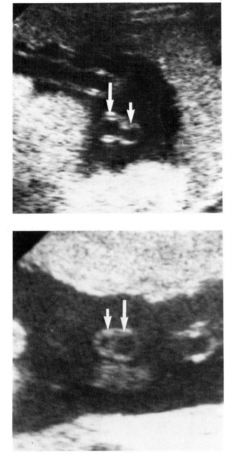

145 and 146. Two-vessel cord; transverse scan of umbilical cord: (*large arrow*) vein; (*small arrow*) artery.

Two-Vessel Cord

One artery and one vein are present owing to aplasia or atrophy of one of the allantoic arteries that would have developed into an umbilical artery. The two-vessel cord is seen in approximately 0.5% to 0.9% of all fetuses. Approximately 10% of these fetuses have other anomalies, often multiple in nature. These include cardiovascular anomalies in approximately 30% and genitourinary anomalies in approximately 28% of deceased infants. There is a 14% mortality rate associated with this condition. Of the deceased infants, 50% had other associated congenital malformations. Of the surviving infants, approximately 4% had associated congenital anomalies, usually of a less critical nature.

Chapter 9

THE UTERUS AND ADNEXAE IN PREGNANCY

The Pregnant Uterus

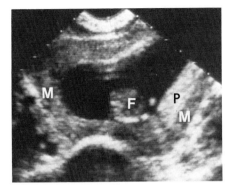

147. Transverse scan of the uterus; homogeneous myometrial texture: (M) myometrium; (P) placenta; (F) fetus.

The normal pregnant uterus has a homogeneous texture throughout the myometrium. The myometrium is of uniform thickness throughout the body and fundus and is usually less than or equal to 1.0 cm in thickness. It is hypoechoic relative to the placenta and hyperechoic relative to the endometrial veins.

The cervix tends to lengthen during pregnancy and varies between 3 and 7 cm from the external to the internal os.

Uterine Contractures

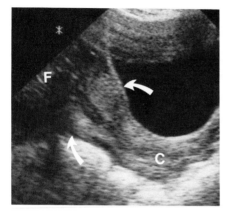

148. Sagittal scan of the uterus; lower uterine segment with circumferential contracture: (C) cervix; (*curved arrows*) contracture; (F) fetus.

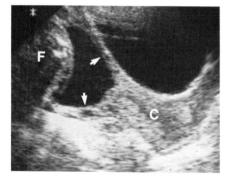

149. Sagittal scan of the uterus; same patient 1 hr later: (C) cervix; (*arrows*) normal myometrium; (F) fetus.

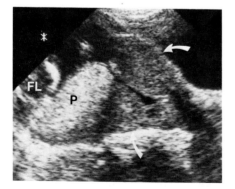

150. Sagittal scan of the uterus: (FL) fetal limb; (P) placenta; (*curved arrows*) circumferential contracture involving myometrium at site of placental attachment. Failure to recognize this may result in a false diagnosis of placenta previa.

Uterine Contractures (*contd.*)

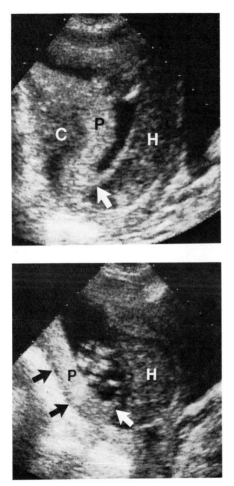

151. Sagittal scan of the uterus; retroplacental contracture: (P) placenta; (*arrow*) elevated margin of placenta; (H) subchorionic hematoma; (C) contracture, which may be misdiagnosed as a retroplacental hematoma.

152. Sagittal scan of the uterus; same patient 1 hr later: (P) placenta; (*white arrow*) elevated margin of placental abruption; (H) subchorionic hematoma; (*black arrows*) normal myometrium.

A uterine contracture can appear throughout pregnancy as a focal thickening of the myometrium or as circumferential myometrial thickening of the lower uterine segment. The term *contracture* distinguishes this phenomenon from the uterine contractions associated with labor. A labor contraction progresses from fundus to cervix, is of shorter duration, and has a higher intensity than a contracture. These may persist unchanged for 45 min or longer. A circumferential contracture in the lower uterine segment may cause the cervix to appear longer than normal and may lead to a false diagnosis of placenta previa. When present beneath the placenta, they may also be mistaken for a retroplacental hematoma or leiomyoma.

Uterine Leiomyoma (Fibroid)

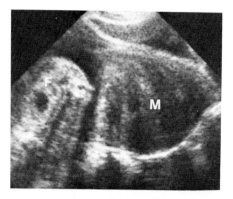

153. Sagittal scan of the uterus; mass in lower uterine segment: (M) mass; (F) fetus. This was a large fibroid or leiomyoma arising from the junction of the lower uterine body and the cervix.

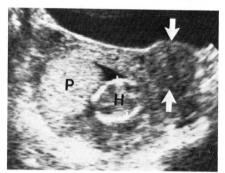

154. Transverse scan of the uterus; mass in myometrium: (*arrows*) mass; (P) placenta; (H) fetal head.

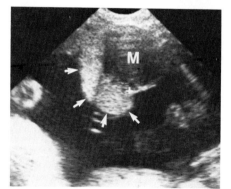

155. Sagittal scan of the uterus; retroplacental mass: (M) mass; (*arrows*) placenta.

Leiomyomas have the same features as in the nongravid uterus. They tend to deform both the serosal and endometrial surfaces of the uterus and are usually hypoechoic relative to the remainder of the myometrium. Due to the effect of estrogen, they tend to enlarge during pregnancy and may infarct and become necrotic. They may interfere with labor. A leiomyoma of the lower uterine segment may interfere with vaginal delivery. A retroplacental leiomyoma may be misinterpreted as a hematoma.

The Incompetent Cervix

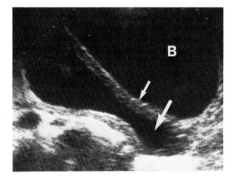

156. Sagittal scan of the cervix: (*large arrow*) membranes and fluid protruding into the endocervical canal; (*short arrow*) anterior wall of cervix.

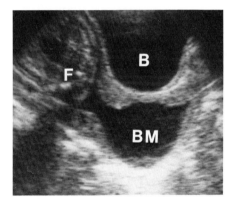

157. Bulging membranes: (F) fetus; (B) bladder; (BM) membranes protruding through the cervix into the vagina.

Patients usually have a history of previous middle trimester painless labor without bleeding or previous cervical injury (i.e., cervical laceration). A cervix of less than 3 cm in length may suggest the diagnosis. Bulging membranes are the diagnostic feature.

Note. An overdistended urinary bladder may compress the anterior and posterior walls of the isthmus area, which may give the false impression of a normal cervix.

Pregnancy Associated with Congenital Uterine Anomalies

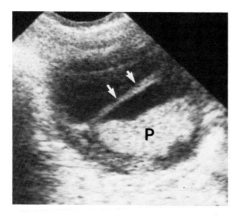

158. Transverse scan of the uterus; congenital intrauterine septum: (*arrows*) septum; (P) placenta.

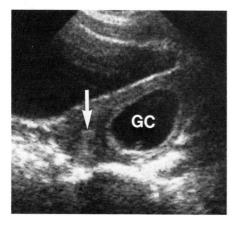

159. Transverse scan of the uterus; bicornuate uterus with anembryonic sac in left cornu: (*arrow*) endometrium of the right cornu; (GC) anembryonic gestational sac.

A *septated uterus* will show a septum bulging into the chorioamniotic cavity. It usually arises from the fundus and extends inferiorly. The fetus can move freely from one side of the septum to the other. This should distinguish it from an amniotic band.

A *bicornuate uterus* may be suggested by an eccentrically located gestational sac and/or by demonstration of a separate endometrial cavity adjacent to the gestational sac.

Corpus Luteum of Pregnancy

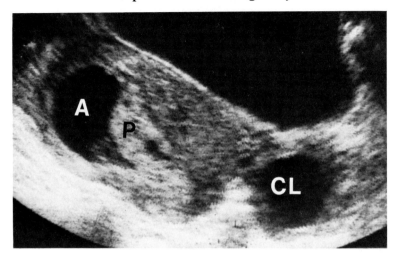

160. Transverse scan of the pelvis; early pregnancy and corpus luteum of pregnancy: (CL) corpus luteum of pregnancy; (P) placenta; (A) amniotic cavity.

If fertilization occurs, the corpus luteum of menstruation enlarges to become the corpus luteum of pregnancy. It is normally present during the first 16 weeks of pregnancy, after which it may resorb. It often appears as a simple cystic mass of 6 cm or less in diameter; however, it may appear septated or contain debris due to hemorrhage. Hemorrhage, rupture, or torsion can cause acute pelvic pain during early pregnancy.

Adnexal Masses in Pregnancy

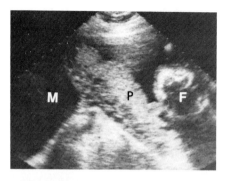

161. Normal pregnancy with a large cyst to the right of and superior to the uterus; transverse scan of the uterus: (M) mass; (P) placenta; (F) fetus.

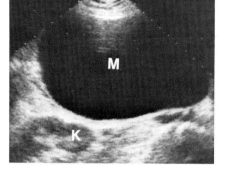

162. Sagittal scan of the mass: (M) mass; (K) kidney.

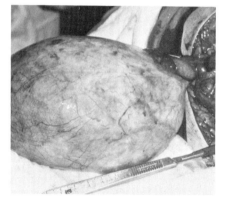

163. Operative specimen; follicular cyst on pathology.

Adnexal masses are occasionally seen during pregnancy. They may be solid or cystic.

The rare coexistent ectopic pregnancy may appear as a cystic, complex, or solid mass with or without free fluid. The quoted incidence varies from 1 in 6,800 pregnancies to 1 in 30,000 pregnancies.

The differential diagnosis of adnexal masses during pregnancy is the same as in the non-pregnant pelvis.

Chapter 10

THE FETUS

The Breech Fetus

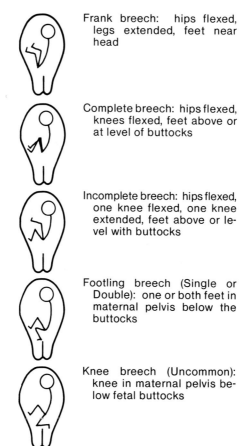

Frank breech: hips flexed, legs extended, feet near head   **164**

Complete breech: hips flexed, knees flexed, feet above or at level of buttocks

Incomplete breech: hips flexed, one knee flexed, one knee extended, feet above or level with buttocks

Footling breech (Single or Double): one or both feet in maternal pelvis below the buttocks

Knee breech (Uncommon): knee in maternal pelvis below fetal buttocks

Fetal lie is the position of the longitudinal axis of the fetus in relation to the longitudinal axis of the uterus (longitudinal, oblique, or transverse). *Fetal presentation* is the fetal part presenting at the birth canal (cephalic, breech, face, foot, hand, or cord).

In the first and second trimesters, the fetus often changes positions during scanning. By first determining the fetal lie, it is possible to identify the right or left side of the fetus and thus to be sure of observing normal fetal anatomy.

In the late third trimester, the fetus usually remains in the same position. The presenting parts should be documented. Attempts should be made to recognize unusual presentations (face, hand, cord) and to detect the different varieties of breech presentation (Fig. 164).

Normal Fetal Head in Early Pregnancy

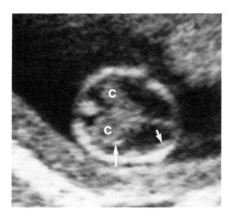

165. Axial scan of fetal head at 13 weeks of gestation: (C) choroid plexuses; (*long arrow*) lateral wall of body of lateral ventricle; (*short arrow*) lateral wall of frontal horn of lateral ventricle.

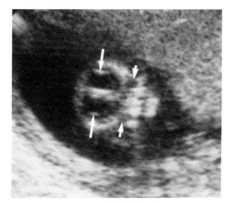

166. Coronal scan of same fetus at 13 weeks of gestation: (*long arrows*) lateral walls of anterior horns of lateral ventricles; (*short arrows*) orbits of fetal skull. (Note that choroid plexus is not present in the frontal horns of the lateral ventricles.)

The lateral ventricles develop from the cerebral vesicles, which appear as two prominent cystic spaces filling much of the cranial vault from approximately 9 to 18 weeks of gestation. Axial scans demonstrate hyperechoic choroid plexuses filling the transverse diameter of the vesicles during this time. After approximately 18 weeks of gestation, the lateral ventricles become more slit-like, and the anatomy closely resembles the structures in the third trimester (see *Fetal Measurements and Calculations*, p. 163).

Lateral Ventricular Ratio

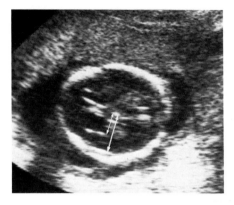

167. Eighteen weeks of gestation; axial scan of fetal head: (*short arrow*) lateral ventricular width (LVW); (*long arrow*) hemispheric width (HW). Lateral ventricular ratio (LVR):

LVR = LVW/HW = 0.55

Normal range for 18 weeks of gestation is 0.42 to 0.62.

The lateral ventricular ratio (LVR) is the ratio of the lateral ventricular width (LVW) to the hemispheric width (HW). The LVW is the distance from the middle of the midline echo to the leading edge of the lateral ventricular wall. The HW is the distance from the middle of the midline echo to the leading edge of the cranial vault.

Lateral Ventricular Ratio (*contd.*)

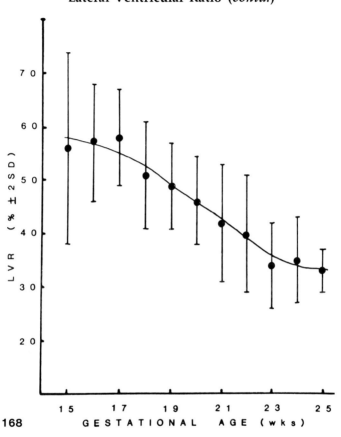

$$LVR = \frac{LVW}{HW} \times 100$$

In the second trimester, the normal LVW should not exceed 1.1 cm. The LVR should normally decrease from a mean of 56% at 15 weeks to 33% at 25 weeks of gestation. The 90th percentile is 74% at 15 weeks and 37% at 25 weeks. Note that ventriculomegaly may exist with a normal LVR. A therapeutic decision must not be based solely on the basis of a single "abnormal" measurement, especially in cases not accompanied by obvious morphological changes. (Graph reproduced with permission from Pretorius, D.H., et al.: *J. Ultrasound Med.* 5:121–124, March 1986, W.B. Saunders, Co.)

Abnormal Head: Anencephaly

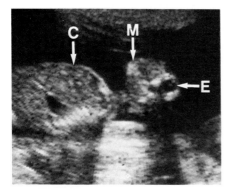

169. Sagittal scan of supine fetus: (M) mandible; (E) eye; (C) anterior chest wall. (*Note.* No evidence of brain tissue cephalad to eye.)

   This condition results from failure of neural tube closure at its cephalad end, between the second and third weeks of development.

   This is the most common congenital defect of the central nervous system (CNS). It occurs in approximately 1 in 1,000 births and more often in female fetuses (4:1). There is a 30-fold risk of recurrence in pregnancies following a previous anencephalic fetus.

   Sonographically, the diagnosis can be made as early as 12 weeks. In every case, there is absence of the cranial vault and of the cerebral hemispheres. The brainstem, base of skull, and orbits are usually present.

   Associated findings include high amniotic fluid and maternal serum alpha-fetoprotein levels, polyhydramnios (40–50% of cases), and spina bifida (50% of cases).

Abnormal Head: Ventriculomegaly

Ventriculomegaly occurs in approximately 2 of 1,000 deliveries. It often accompanies a neural tube defect. It may result from an obstruction in the cerebrospinal fluid pathway (obstructive hydrocephalus) or may result from atrophy of the brain parenchyma with subsequent passive dilatation of the ventricles (hydrocephalus *ex vacuo*).

When ventricular dilatation is gross or associated with an enlarged head, the abnormality is obvious. Accurate detection of ventriculomegaly in early pregnancy is more difficult but possible with careful scanning. Early sonographic manifestations of ventriculomegaly include the following:

1. Dilatation of the occipital horn and trigone, which is the first sign to occur between 20 and 25 weeks of gestation. When this is seen, follow-up studies are mandatory.

2. Shrinking of the choroid plexus because of increased intraventricular pressure. Ultrasonography demonstrates a small choroid plexus, which fails to fill the transverse diameter of the body of the lateral ventricle.

3. Displacement of the medial wall of the body of the lateral ventricle toward the midline. In the normal ventricle, the medial wall is usually not seen. It becomes more apparent when the ventricle is dilated.

Serial determination of the lateral ventricle ratio (LVR) may also be helpful. If the LVR fails to decrease between 15 and 25 weeks of gestation, then ventriculomegaly must be suspected.

Abnormal Head: Ventriculomegaly (*contd.*)

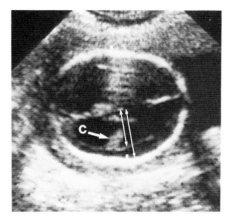

170. Ventriculomegaly at 19 weeks of gestation; axial scan of fetal head: (*short arrow*) lateral ventricular width (LVW); (C) choroid plexus; (*long arrow*) hemispheric width (HW). Lateral ventricular ratio (LVR):

$$LVR = LVW/HW = 0.75$$

Normal range for 19 weeks is 0.40 to 0.58.

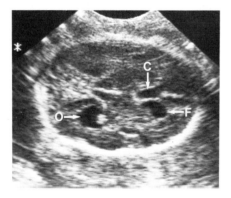

171. Mild to moderate ventriculomegaly; axial scan of fetal head at 30 weeks of gestation: (O) trigone of lateral ventricle; (F) frontal horn of lateral ventricle; (C) cavum septi pellucidi (normal). (*Note.* This was unilateral ventriculomegaly due to congenital stenosis of the right foramen of Monro.)

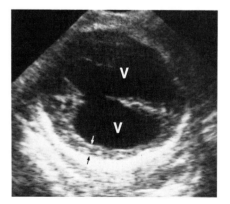

172. Advanced ventriculomegaly; axial scan of fetal head at 36 weeks of gestation: (V) grossly enlarged lateral ventricle; (*arrows*) thin brain parenchyma.

Abnormal Head: Hydranencephaly

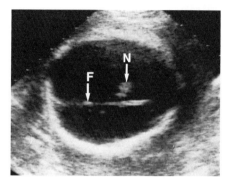

173. Axial scan of fetal head at 30 weeks of gestation: (F) falx; (N) nubbin of brain tissue. No other brain tissue is visible in this section. (*Note.* Biparietal diameter was appropriate for gestational age.)

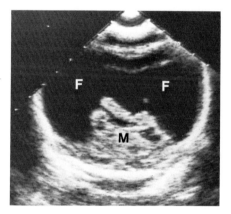

174. Coronal scan of neonatal brain through the anterior fontanelle shortly after birth: (M) midbrain; (F) fluid filling the supratentorial compartment of the cranial vault. (*Note.* Only a small rim of cortical brain was present in the occipital area.)

This is a rare condition of obscure etiology. Hypotheses include vascular occlusion and infections, resulting in nondevelopment of the cerebral hemispheres, which are replaced by fluid-filled cavities. The characteristic sonographic findings are the following:

1. normal cranial vault and head size;
2. falx often but not always absent;
3. absent cerebral hemispheres, except for portions of the occipital lobes; typically, the basal ganglia and the brainstem as well as the cerebellum are preserved;
4. absence of other associated anomalies.

Massive hydrocephalus is difficult to distinguish from hydranencephaly.

Abnormal Head: Encephalocele

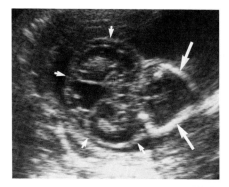

175. Axial scan of fetal head at 28 weeks of gestation: (*long arrows*) small deformed cranial vault; (*short arrows*) meninges and brain tissue herniated through defect along posterior aspect of cranial vault.

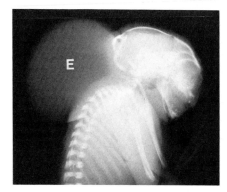

176. Lateral radiograph of specimen after delivery: (E) large encephalocele along posterior aspect of small cranial vault.

An encephalocele represents a defect in the cranial vault through which protrude intracranial contents. The incidence is 1 in 2,000 births. The defect is occipital in 75% of cases, frontoethmoidal in 13%, and parietal in 12%.

The sonographic appearance is that of a cystic and/or solid mass along the external aspect of the cranial vault. The defect in the cranial vault may also be seen. Associated abnormalities include polyhydramnios and ventriculomegaly. Care must be taken to distinguish an encephalocele from a cystic hygroma or a hemangioma.

The Normal Fetal Spine

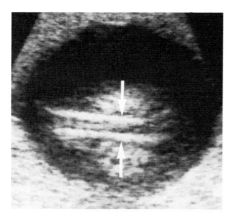

177. Coronal scan of fetal spine: (*arrows*) normal parallel posterior elements of the thoracolumbar spine.

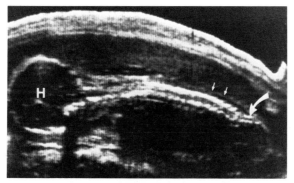

178. Sagittal scan of fetal spine: (H) head; (*short arrows*) skin surface of lumbar area; (*curved arrow*) sacrum.

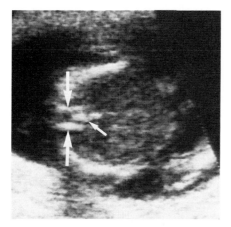

179. Axial scan of fetal lumbar spine: (*long arrows*) normal posterior spinal elements; (*short arrow*) normal ossified vertebral body.

The Normal Fetal Spine (*contd.*)

Demonstration of a normal fetal spine between 16 and 20 weeks of gestation is important because of therapeutic implications in the case of a spinal defect. Careful scanning should include the following:

1. A coronal scan through the long axis, demonstrating the posterior spinal elements as two parallel lines. There is normally mild divergence or widening in the cervical area.

2. A sagittal scan through the long axis, demonstrating the skin and subcutaneous tissue along the posterior aspect of the fetal back.

3. Axial scans at various levels (cervical down to sacral) at 90° to the long axis of the fetal spine. The ossified posterior elements of the spine (the laminae) appear as two parallel lines. The vertebral body appears as a single hyperechoic focus anterior to the laminae.

Spina Bifida

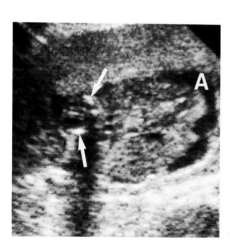

180. Gestation, 29 weeks; coronal scan through thoraco-lumbar fetal spine: (*arrows*) divergence of posterior spinal elements.

181. Gestation, 29 weeks; axial scan through lumbar spine of the same fetus: (*arrows*) divergent posterior spinal elements; (A) ascites due to Rh isoimmunization.

A spina bifida represents a defect in the bony neural canal (usually situated posteriorly). It results from failure of fusion of the neural arches during development.

Sonographic signs of spina bifida are the following:

1. Widening of the posterior spinal elements compared to levels cephalad and/or caudal to the area of interest (detected on coronal and axial scanning);

2. Divergence of the posterior spinal elements as demonstrated on axial scans. The posterior elements diverge posteriorly instead of forming two parallel lines.

Meningocele–Myelomeningocele

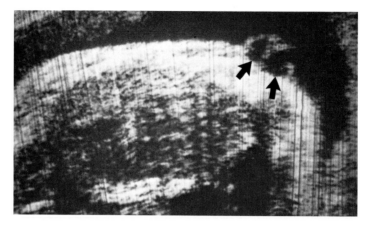

182. Sagittal scan of fetal back: (*arrows*) lower lumbar myelomeningocele.

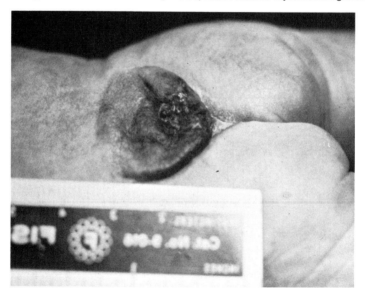

183. Picture of myelomeningocele shortly after birth.

When there is herniation of the meninges and/or neural tissue through the bony defect, a meningocele or myelomeningocele is formed. The meningeal protrusion appears as a cystic mass, with a solid component if it contains neural tissue. Common associated malformations include ventriculomegaly.

Anencephaly, encephalocele, spina bifida, meningocele, and myelomeningocele form the spectrum of neural tube defects that constitute the majority of fetal malformations; 90% of cases are the first occurrence in the family, whereas 10% occur in families with a previous child affected.

Diastematomyelia

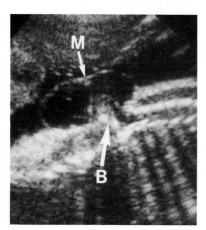

184. Gestation, 37 weeks; coronal scan of lower thoracic fetal spine: (B) bone septum in spinal canal; (*arrows*) divergence of posterior elements.

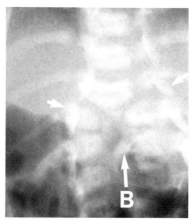

185. Gestation, 37 weeks; sagittal scan of lower thoracic fetal spine: (B) bone septum in spinal canal; (M) meningocele sac.

186. Post delivery; radiograph of thoracolumbar spine: (B) bone septum in spinal canal; (*arrows*) divergence of posterior elements.

Diastematomyelia implies splitting of the spinal cord by a fibrous or bony septum that courses in a sagittal plane across the spinal canal. If the septum is ossified, it may be detected on radiography and prenatal ultrasound (Figs. 184–186). Diastematomyelia may or may not be associated with a myelomeningocele. The patient in Figs. 184–186 had both diastematomyelia and a myelomeningocele.

The Normal Thorax: The Heart

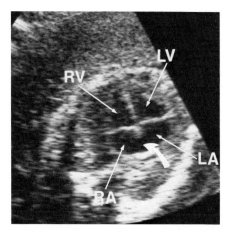

187. Four-chamber view of the fetal heart at 27 weeks of gestation: (RV) right ventricle; (LV) left ventricle; (LA) left atrium; (RA) right atrium; (*curved arrow*) the apparent opening in the interatrial septum represents the foramen ovale.

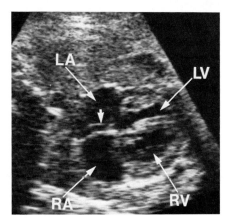

188. Four-chamber view of the fetal heart at 35 weeks of gestation: (LA) left atrium; (LV) left ventricle; (RV) right ventricle; (RA) right atrium; (*arrow*) normal membrane covering the foramen ovale of the interatrial septum.

The fetal thorax is slightly smaller in diameter compared to the abdomen. Routinely visualized structures include the ribs and chest wall and the lungs and heart. In sagittal and coronal scans, the diaphragm is often visible as a thin hypoechoic structure (see *The Normal Abdomen,* p. 133).

In the late second and third trimesters, it is possible to obtain detailed two-dimensional images of the cardiac structures in multiple planes. Present techniques allow detection of positional abnormalities, large intracardiac defects, and rhythm abnormalities.

Indications for Fetal Echocardiography

Detailed fetal cardiac assessment is indicated in the following circumstances:

1. A history of congenital heart disease in the mother or previous child indicates a higher risk in subsequent fetuses.

2. Selected maternal disorders predispose to congenital heart disease or cardiac malfunction. These include Rh isoimmunization, maternal diabetes mellitus, connective tissue disorders, storage diseases, and phenylketonuria (PKU).

3. Certain teratogens, drugs, and infectious processes can cause congenital heart diseases. These include rubella infection, exposure to phenytoin sodium, alcohol, lithium, oral contraceptives. Certain antihypertensive agents and tocolytic agents (to inhibit premature labor) can alter fetal cardiac rhythm and rate.

4. Certain fetal abnormalities predispose to cardiac anomalies and arrhythmias. Fetuses with one anomaly often have another. Fetuses with abnormal growth have greater risk. There is a high incidence of cardiac anomalies with trisomy 21, 18, or 13. Twenty percent of fetuses with an arrhythmia have major structural congenital heart disease.

The Abnormal Thorax: The Abnormal Heart

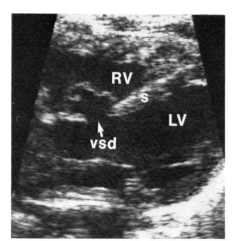

189. Ventricular septal defect long-axis view of heart: (RV) right ventricular cavity; (LV) left ventricular cavity; (S) interventricular septum; (vsd) ventricular septal defect of membranous portion of ventricular septum.

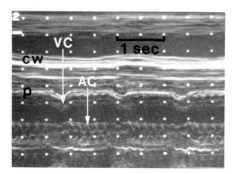

190. Atrioventricular block: M-mode scan of heart; (CW) chest wall of fetus; (P) pericardium; (VC) ventricular contraction; (AC) atrial contraction. (*Note.* There are six atrial contractions for every single ventricular contraction. This constitutes a 6:1 atrioventricular block.)

Congenital heart disease occurs in more than 0.01% of live births and 10% of stillbirths. Cardiac arrhythmias occur in 1% of newborns; the exact frequency in fetuses is not known. A cardiac anomaly should be suspected if the paired chambers or the great vessels (i.e., aorta and pulmonary artery) are disproportionate in size. It is possible to diagnose larger anatomic defects, such as atrial septal defect, ventricular septal defect, and a single ventricle.

Arrhythmias are best diagnosed and documented with M-mode scans. The atrial and ventricular rhythms may be simultaneously sampled by directing the sound beam diagonally through one ventricle and the opposite atrium (see above example).

The Abnormal Thorax: Pleural Effusion

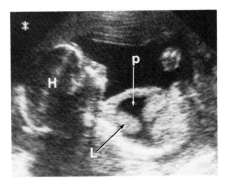

191. Sagittal scan of the fetal head and chest at 29 weeks of gestation: (H) head; (P) pleural effusion; (L) left lung.

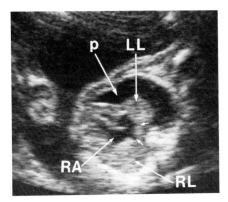

192. Axial scan of the same fetal chest at 29 weeks of gestation: (P) pleural effusion; (LL) left lung; (RL) right lung; (RA) right atrium of heart; (*small arrows*) pulmonary veins entering the left atrium. (Note the foramen ovale between the left and right atrium. This pleural effusion gradually resorbed during pregnancy. A cause was not found in postnatal investigations of the neonate.)

A small to moderate pleural effusion will appear as a fluid collection enveloping a portion of the fetal lung. This condition causes little problem in diagnosis. However, the fluid collection may become large and cause gross displacement of surrounding structures, in which case a differentiation from other conditions, such as diaphragmatic hernia or cystadenomatoid malformation, may be difficult.

The Abnormal Thorax: Cystic Adenomatoid
Malformation of the Lung

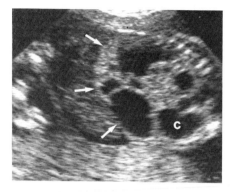

193. Long-axis coronal scan of the fetal chest: (*arrows*) eventrated diaphragmatic surface; (C) one of several cysts in the large mass that fills the fetal chest.

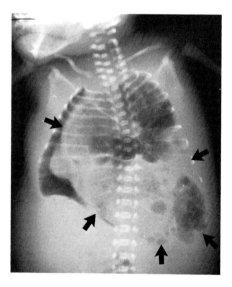

194. Postmortem radiograph of the chest. (*arrows*) large cystic adenomatoid mass filling the chest and causing caudal displacement and eventration of the diaphragm.

This rare malformation of the lung is characterized by cysts of various sizes in the fetal thorax. The cysts may be single or multiple. One lobe, one lung, or both lungs may be affected. Associated findings include polyhydramnios and hydrops fetalis.

Abnormal Abdominal Wall: Omphalocele

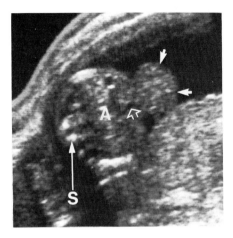

195. Transverse scan of fetal abdomen at 23 weeks of gestation: (A) abdominal cavity at the level of the liver; (*short arrows*) smooth-walled mass (omphalocele) protruding from the anterior abdominal wall; (*open arrow*) umbilical vein entering the base of the omphalocele; (S) spine.

Omphalocele represents a defect in the anterior abdominal wall at the site of umbilical cord insertion. Bowel and liver tissue may herniate through the defect into a sac that protrudes outside the abdominal cavity. Occasionally, the peritoneal sac, which comprises the wall of the sac, may rupture, making distinction from gastroschisis more difficult.

The incidence is approximately 1 in 5,800 births. Two-thirds of patients have other anomalies as well: urogenital, 40%; chromosomal, 30%; cardiovascular, 20%; and neurological, 4%.

Abnormal Abdominal Wall: Gastroschisis

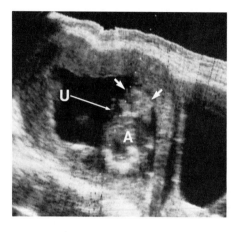

196. Axial scan of the fetal abdomen at 18 weeks of gestation: (A) abdominal cavity; (U) umbilical cord; (*arrows*) irregularly marginated mass attached to the anterior abdominal wall to the right of the umbilical cord insertion. This represents herniated loops of small bowel.

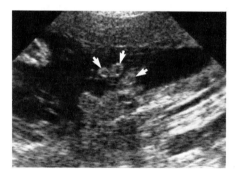

197. Scan through the pregnant uterus at 35 weeks of gestation in the same fetus: (*arrows*) separate loops of small bowel floating freely in amniotic fluid outside the fetal abdomen.

This anterior abdominal wall defect is one-third as common as an omphalocele. It differs from omphalocele by the following features:

1. The defect is usually on the right side.
2. The umbilical cord inserts normally into the anterior abdominal wall.
3. There is invariably evisceration of the small bowel, but sometimes of the stomach and colon as well. Malrotation is a constant finding.
4. The herniated content is not covered by a membrane.
5. Associated major malformations are uncommon.

Polyhydramnios and increased alpha-fetoprotein in amniotic fluid are found in both omphalocele and gastroschisis. Early diagnosis, prompt surgical correction, and improved postsurgical care have lowered the mortality rate, which has been high.

The Normal Abdomen

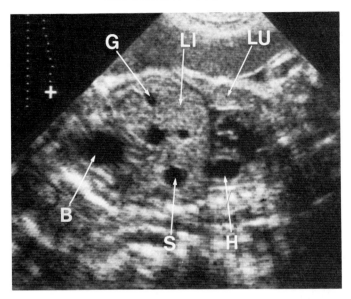

198. Coronal scan of chest and abdomen: (G) gallbladder; (LI) liver; (LU) lung (right); (H) heart (left ventricle); (S) stomach; (B) bladder; the diaphragm is the thin hypoechoic zone between the liver and right lung.

Scanning the normal fetal abdomen usually allows detection of the following structures: the abdominal wall; the insertion of the umbilical cord; the liver; the kidneys; the stomach; the bladder; and vascular structures, such as the inferior vena cava, aorta, umbilical vein, and portal veins. The vascular landmarks are important in acquiring the appropriate axial scan for abdominal diameter and circumference measurements (see *Fetal Measurements and Calculations,* p. 165).

The Normal Fetal Urinary System

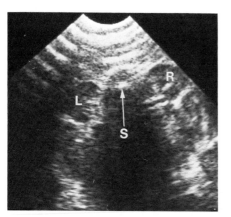

199. Axial scan of the fetal back and abdomen: (L) left kidney; (S) spine; (R) right kidney.

200. Coronal scan through the flank of a fetus: (S) sinus echoes from the central portion of the kidney; (C) cortex in the upper pole of the kidney; (PS) psoas muscle.

In 90% of pregnancies, the fetal kidneys are seen between 17 and 22 weeks of gestation. Earlier visualization requires optimal conditions. The ratio of maximum kidney circumference to fetal abdominal circumference is fairly uniform throughout gestation and is approximately 0.30.

The fetal kidney normally appears as a reniform structure with a smooth outline. Its cortex is less echogenic than the liver and the central sinus complex. The renal pyramids appear as small hypoechoic areas distributed uniformly throughout the renal medulla. The urinary bladder can be detected in the second trimester as a cystic structure between the iliac wings. It may be empty at the time of scanning, and a repeat scan in 30 to 45 min may demonstrate filling.

Transient Hydronephrosis

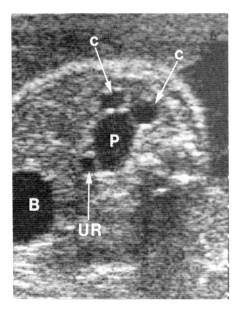

201. Oblique scan through the fetal abdomen at 35 weeks of gestation, demonstrating moderate hydronephrosis: (C) calyx, fluid-filled and dilated; (P) renal pelvis; (UR) proximal ureter; (B) bladder.

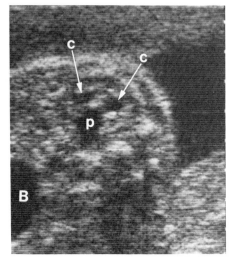

202. Oblique scan through the fetal abdomen 1 min later, demonstrating a decrease in the hydronephrosis: (C) calyx; (P) renal pelvis; (B) bladder. After birth, there was no evidence of hydronephrosis.

Transient Hydronephrosis (*contd.*)

Hydronephrosis is dilatation of the intrarenal collecting system, and this may reflect obstructive or nonobstructive conditions *in utero*. Hydronephrosis may be unilateral or bilateral; it may begin at any stage of pregnancy after the kidneys begin to function; and it may vary in severity. Hydronephrosis is the most common abnormality of the fetal and neonatal genitourinary tract.

A diagnostic problem in obstetric ultrasound involves the presence of mild to moderate hydronephrosis. This may represent a permanent obstruction at one of several points in the urinary system, or it may reflect a transient phenomenon. These transient phenomena include the following:

1. Transient obstruction (full fetal bladder).
2. Increased urine production (maternal and fetal diuresis due to fluid loading before the ultrasound scan).
3. Vesicoureteric reflux.
4. A normal variant.

The distinction among these and between permanent obstructions often requires repeat scans *in utero* and/or after birth.

Obstructive Hydronephrosis

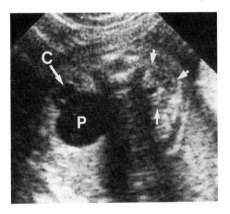

203. Axial scan of fetal back and abdomen at 32 weeks of gestation: (C) dilated calyx; (P) dilated renal pelvis; (*arrows*) normal right kidney.

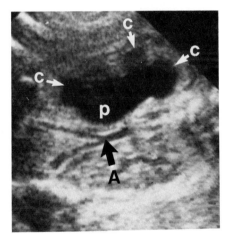

204. Left coronal scan of the same fetus: (C) dilated calyces; (A) distal abdominal aorta and bifurcation into common iliac arteries; (P) dilated renal pelvis. The ureter could not be visualized. Postnatal examinations revealed a ureteropelvic junction stenosis.

Permanent partial obstruction can cause mild to severe hydronephrosis *in utero*. The most common cause of unilateral obstruction is a stenosis at the uretero-pelvic junction. Other causes include stenosis at the ureterovesical junction, ureteroceles, and bladder outlet obstruction (most commonly due to posterior urethral valves in boys).

Multicystic Dysplastic Kidney

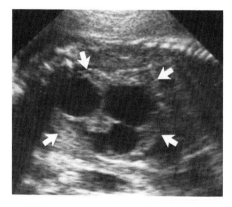

205. Long-axis scan of right kidney: (*arrows*) large mass replacing fetal kidney. (*Note.* Mass has several cysts and hyperechoic "solid" material within it. The other kidney was normal.)

Urinary tract obstruction during nephrogenesis accounts for 90% of dysplastic kidneys. Multicystic dysplasia appears to result from obstruction by ureteropelvic atresia occurring between 8 and 10 weeks of gestation. It is most often unilateral, and it is the most common palpable abdominal mass in the neonate. Pathologically, the entire affected kidney is replaced by single or multiple cysts that do not communicate with one another. There is usually no appreciable normal renal tissue. Hydronephrosis of the contralateral kidney may be seen in 10% to 20% of cases. After birth, recent consensus is to observe and follow up the multicystic kidney with serial ultrasound examinations. These usually involute spontaneously after a period of time.

Polycystic Kidneys: Infantile Type

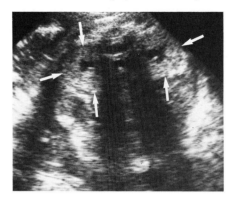

206. Axial scan through fetal back: (*arrows*) both kidneys consist of hyperechoic material throughout the parenchyma. (*Note.* Mildly dilated collecting system within each kidney.)

Infantile polycystic kidneys result from a genetic defect in nephrogenesis transmitted as autosomal recessive. There is a 25% risk of recurrence with each pregnancy if both parents have the abnormal gene.

Both kidneys show symmetrical enlargement, with proliferation and dilatation of tubules extending into the entire cortex. The kidney circumference/abdominal circumference ratio is often more than 0.50.

Sonographically, the enlarged kidneys appear more echogenic than normal, with loss of the tissue plane between liver and kidney and loss of corticomedullary distinction. The increased echogenicity comes from the multiple dilated tubules, which are not large enough to resolve as separate fluid-filled structures.

Potter's Syndrome

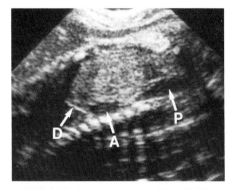

207. Long-axis scan of fetal abdomen: (D) diaphragm; (A) adrenal gland; (P) psoas muscle. (*Note.* No amniotic fluid present. No kidney in renal fossa.)

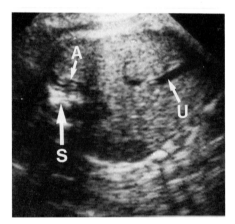

208. Axial scan of fetal abdomen: (S) spine; (A) adrenal gland; (L) liver; (U) umbilical vein. (*Note.* No kidney in renal fossa.)

The typical syndrome is characterized by

renal agenesis;
oligohydramnios or anhydramnios;
pulmonary hypoplasia; and
characteristic facies.

The "oligohydramnios–hypoplastic lung" complex is also seen in other genitourinary malformations, such as renal hypoplasia, cystic dysplasia, posterior urethral valves, and prune-belly syndrome. This is also seen in a few cases of autosomal recessive polycystic kidney disease.

If renal agenesis is suspected *in utero,* a furosemide challenge test can be performed. Failure to visualize the urinary bladder on serial scans suggests absence of functioning kidneys.

Bladder Outlet Obstruction

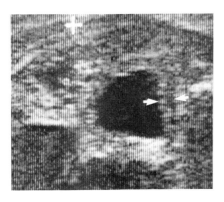

209. Sagittal scan of fetal bladder: (*arrows*) thickened bladder wall.

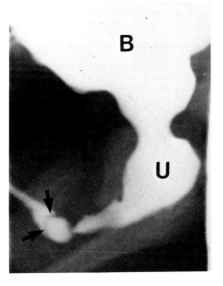

210. Voiding cystourethrogram after birth: (B) bladder; (U) dilated urethra; (*arrows*) congenital valves causing obstruction in anterior urethra.

In male fetuses, urethral obstruction is most commonly due to *posterior* urethral valves. Figures 209 and 210 show an example of an obstructing *anterior* valve, which is a much rarer abnormality. Other less frequent causes include urethral diverticulum and ectopic ureterocele.

The fetal urinary bladder normally appears as a cystic structure without an appreciable wall thickness. Long-standing incomplete outlet obstruction results in the thickening of the wall, which then becomes visible as a distinct hypoechoic rim of tissue. When this is seen *in utero,* a bladder outlet obstruction should be suspected, and further investigations should be contemplated after birth.

Prune-Belly Syndrome

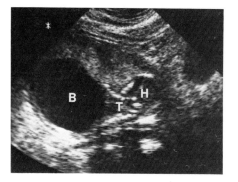

211. Sagittal scan of uterus at 19 weeks of gestation: (H) fetal head; (T) thoracic cavity; (B) cystic mass filling abdominal cavity (distended urinary bladder). (*Note.* Anhydramnios.)

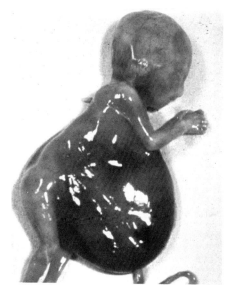

212. Photograph of specimen after delivery. (*Note.* Large protuberant abdomen due to grossly distended urinary bladder.)

Some authors prefer the term "urethral obstruction malformation complex," implying urethral obstruction as the fundamental pathological event.

The condition consists of cryptorchidism; agenesis of abdominal wall musculature; and megaureters. There is nearly always bladder outlet obstruction, often due to urethral anomalies, such as atresia, stenosis, valves, or diverticulum.

Sonographically, the protruding fetal abdomen may be filled with numerous cystic lesions, representing the tortuous dilated ureters and dilated bladder. Associated findings are fetal ascites, hypoplastic lungs, and oligohydramnios.

Duodenal Obstruction

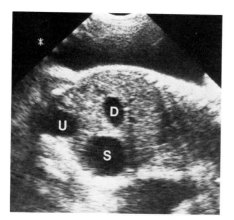

213. Coronal scan of fetal abdomen: (U) urinary bladder; (S) stomach dilated; (D) duodenum, dilated. (*Note.* Polyhydramnios with amniotic fluid between uterine wall and fetal abdomen.

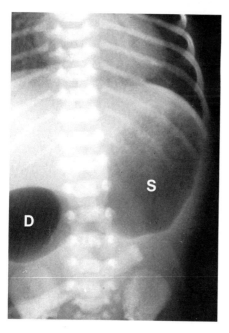

214. Radiograph of neonatal abdomen 1 day after birth: (S) dilated stomach; (D) dilated duodenum.

This is a relatively common obstructive lesion of the fetal gastrointestinal tract; 33% of cases are associated with Down's syndrome. It may be found in conjunction with esophageal atresia, and this is usually a lethal combination after birth.

The obstruction most often involves the second part of the duodenum, resulting in a dilated fluid-filled stomach and duodenal segment proximal to the atresia. They appear sonographically as two cystic masses corresponding to the "double bubble" following birth.

Gallstones

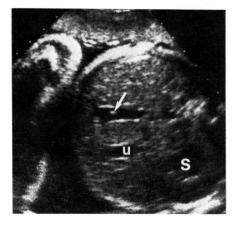

215. Axial scan of the fetal abdomen: (*arrow*) small calculus inside gallbladder; (U) umbilical portion of left portal vein; (S) stomach.

The gallbladder appears as a small cystic structure lying on the right side of the abdomen, in the same axial plane as the umbilical vein. Rarely, prenatal scans may demonstrate apparent calculi within the fetal gallbladder. These may resorb and disappear in the early neonatal period and cause no clinical abnormalities.

Genitalia: Normal

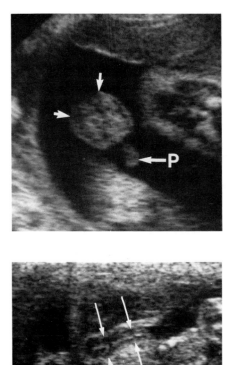

216. Normal male genitalia; (P) penis; (*arrows*) scrotum containing two testicles.

217. Normal female genitalia. Oblique scan through the buttocks demonstrating a portion of the female genitalia: (*arrows*) margin of the labia majora. The *white line* is the interface of the labia.

In the third trimester, it is possible in most fetuses to visualize the external genitalia and thus confirm the sex of the fetus. However, we specifically scan this area only when there is a medical indication (e.g., possible X-linked chromosomal abnormality or possible bladder outlet obstruction due to posterior urethral valves in a male fetus). Errors in interpretation may arise when swollen labia or the umbilical cord mimic male genitalia in the female fetus.

Even before the testicles descend into the scrotum, it is possible in male fetuses to detect the normal penis with a fair degree of confidence in early pregnancy (as early as 14 weeks of gestation).

Abnormal Genitalia: Hydrocele

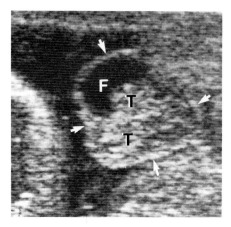

218. Oblique scan through scrotum: (*arrows*) scrotal sac; (F) fluid of hydrocele adjacent to one testicle; (T) testicles.

The normal fetal scrotum is usually first seen at 25 weeks of gestation as an ovoid anterior soft tissue mass projecting from the fetal rump.

Hydrocele has been diagnosed *in utero* as a fluid collection in the scrotum, surrounding the echogenic testes. It results from a persistent processus vaginallis, which normally closes late in fetal life or even after birth. Therefore, hydrocele is probably not significant if found *in utero.*

The Normal Limbs

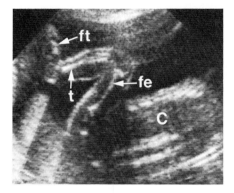

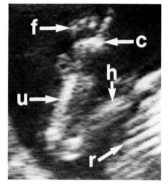

219. Sagittal scan of a supine fetus: (ft) foot; (t) tibia; (fe) femur; (C) chest.

220. (F) fingers; (C) carpal bones; (U) ulna; (h) humerus; (r) ribs.

The *primary* ossification centers of the appendicular skeleton can be detected in the first trimester. The two *secondary* ossification centers commonly seen prenatally are those of the distal femur and proximal tibia. A few general rules are helpful: (a) serial femur length measurements are most helpful in detecting short-limbed dysplasias; and (b) the distal radius and ulna and tibia and fibula end at the same point. If one bone is hypoplastic, it does not end at the same distal level as the other. This is helpful in assessing possible limb reduction. In a high-risk population, the following questions have to be answered:

1. Are all the long bones present?
2. Is the femur length normal for gestational age?
3. Does the femur appear to grow normally on serial scans?
4. Is there any limb reduction defect?
5. Is there any fracture?
6. Is the bone brightness (echogenicity) normal?
7. Is there any other fetal anomaly?

By systematically answering these questions, certain skeletal dysplasias may be diagnosed prenatally in the second and third trimesters. We must remember, however, that the role of ultrasound remains limited by technical factors and by the fact that certain skeletal dysplasias may not manifest themselves *in utero*.

Dwarfism: Thanatophoric Dwarfism

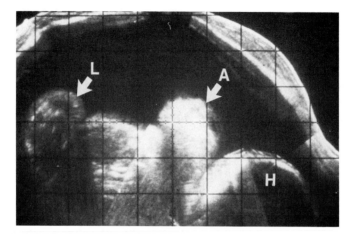

221. Thanatophoric dwarfism. Sagittal scan of the uterus: (H) fetal head; (A) short arm; (L) short leg. (*Note.* Marked hydramnios.)

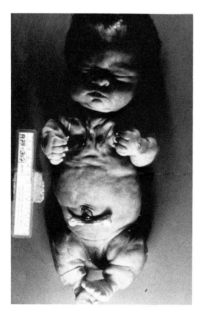

222. Thanatophoric dwarfism. Picture of specimen shortly after birth. Note the very short arms and legs.

This lethal condition is a dominant mutation affecting predominantly male fetuses. The thorax is small, and the limbs are markedly short throughout the entire gestation. In the most common form of dwarfism (achondroplasia), however, the short limbs may only become manifest after 20 weeks of gestation. Normal bone lengths before 20 weeks of gestation do not rule out achondroplasia.

Trisomy 18: Edward's Syndrome

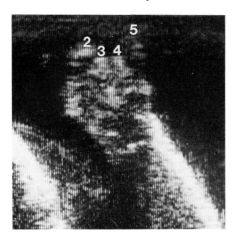

223. Scan of fetal hand: (2, 5) second and fifth fingers are extended; (3, 4) third and fourth fingers are flexed.

224. Picture of neonatal hand shortly after birth. Note the extended second and fifth fingers and the flexed third and fourth fingers.

The characteristic finding is flexion deformity of the third and fourth fingers; the first, second, and fifth fingers are partially extended.

Associated features are low fetal weight and club foot.

Ovarian Cyst

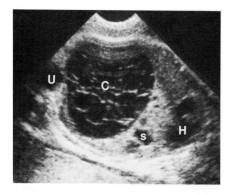

225. Coronal scan of fetal abdomen: (U) urinary bladder; (C) theca lutein cyst filling abdominal cavity; (S) stomach; (H) heart.

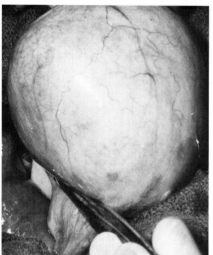

226. Picture of mass at surgery. (*Note.* Large theca lutein cyst with a smooth surface.)

Ovarian cysts are rarely seen *in utero.* Only a few sporadic cases have been reported in the literature.

This example of a theca lutein cyst appears sonographically as a multiseptated cystic mass filling the entire fetal abdomen. Ovarian cysts occur more commonly in fetuses born of diabetic mothers. When seen in association with polyhydramnios and signs of fetal macrosomia, a glucose tolerance test should be performed. It is postulated that ovarian cysts develop in the fetus in response to the effect of maternal human chorionic gonadotropin, which is often produced in increased amounts in gestational diabetes. Following birth, serial scans should be performed to monitor the cyst, which usually regresses spontaneously over a period of time.

Fetus of Diabetic Mother

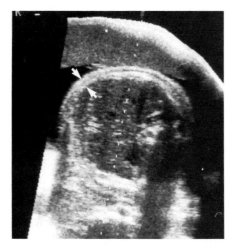

227. Axial scan of fetal abdomen: (*arrows*) subcutaneous fat.

Diabetes mellitus is a common complication of pregnancy. Overt diabetes occurs in 1 of 200 pregnancies, whereas gestational diabetes occurs in 5 of 200 pregnancies. The disease often produces deleterious effects on the fetus, which shows a higher incidence of congenital structural malformations and growth disorders than the general population. Common congenital anomalies include neural tube, cardiovascular, gastrointestinal, and genitourinary malformations. Growth disorders include macrosomia for diabetic mothers of classes A, B, and C and intrauterine growth retardation for those classes associated with vasculopathy, namely classes D, F, H, R, and T. Fetal macrosomia is characterized by thickened soft tissues (abdominal wall more than 5 mm in thickness) and increased fetal weight, which may exceed the 95th percentile for a given period of gestation. A thickened placenta and polyhydramnios are also often present.

Turner's Syndrome

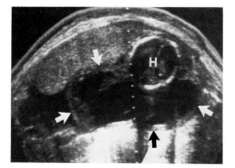

228. Axial scan of fetal head: (H) head; (*arrows*) large septated cystic hygroma along posterior aspect of head.

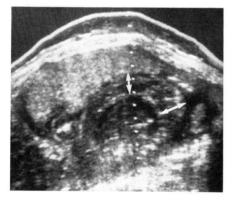

229. Axial scan of fetal abdomen: (*arrows*) marked subcutaneous lymphedema.

Turner's syndrome is a chromosomal disorder wherein the fetus has a 45X karyotype instead of 46XX. The incidence is approximately 1 in 2,500 newborn girls but is higher in spontaneous abortuses (9–29%). Somatic malformations affect tissues of mesodermal origin (i.e., the skeleton and connective tissue). Cervical cystic hygroma, generalized subcutaneous lymphedema, ascites, and polyhydramnios may be detected during prenatal sonograms as early as 18 weeks of gestation.

Fetal Hydrops (Hydrops Fetalis)

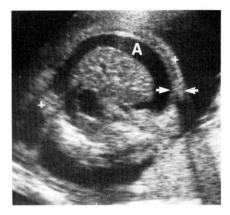

230. Axial scan of fetal abdomen with advanced hydrops. (A) ascites surrounding the liver; (*arrows*) thickness of abdominal wall (11 mm); (+) abdominal diameter. This was nonimmune hydrops in a fetus with Down's syndrome.

The condition is characterized by generalized soft tissue edema (anasarca), usually associated with ascites, pleural effusion, and pericardial effusions.

The most common cause is Rh isoimmunization; however, there are more than 40 other conditions that may produce fetal hydrops. Certain conditions, such as paroxysmal atrial tachycardia, fetal anemia, or congestive heart failure, can be treated *in utero*.

The role of ultrasound is as follows:

1. To detect hydrops, to evaluate its severity, and to follow its evolution. Fetal soft tissue thickening is present if this exceeds 5 mm as measured in the abdominal wall.

2. To detect associated fetal structural anomalies that may be present in 25% to 50% of cases. They include skeletal dysplasias, genitourinary and gastrointestinal malformations, CNS defects or infections, and mediastinal and abdominal tumors.

3. To evaluate placental thickness and morphology. Chorangioma if large may lead to hydrops.

4. To guide amniocentesis and *in utero* transfusion.

Cystic Hygroma

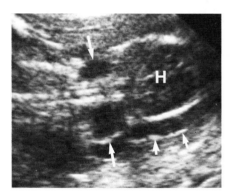

231. Sagittal scan through fetal head at 18 weeks of gestation: (O) occipital bone of skull; (*long arrows*) cystic hygroma enveloping fetal skull; (*short arrows*) cystic hygroma along anterior aspect of neck.

232. Coronal scan through the fetal head and neck in the same fetus: (H) head; (*short arrows*) cystic hygroma enveloping fetal head; (*long arrows*) cystic hygroma along the sides of the neck.

This congenital malformation of the lymphatic system occurs in 1 of 6,000 pregnancies resulting from lymphatic obstruction. It is seen most commonly in association with chromosomal abnormalities, such as Turner's syndrome, Noonan's syndrome, Down's syndrome, and various trisomies.

Ninety-five percent of cystic hygromas are found in the neck; other sites are the axilla and groin.

Ultrasound usually demonstrates a cystic mass, which may be septated, projecting from the neck, axillae, or groin. The wall of the cyst may be thin or may show a focal mass of solid tissue. It may be difficult to differentiate from a hemangioma, teratoma, or neural tube defect. Associated findings, such as placental thickening and fetal hydrops, are helpful in making the diagnosis of cystic hygroma.

Sacrococcygeal Teratoma

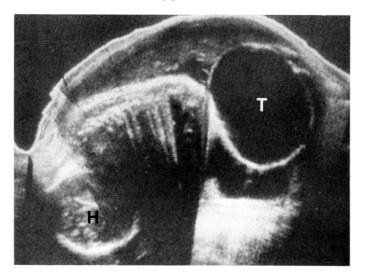

233. Sagittal scan through the fetal back: (H) head; (T) cystic mass adjacent to sacrum.

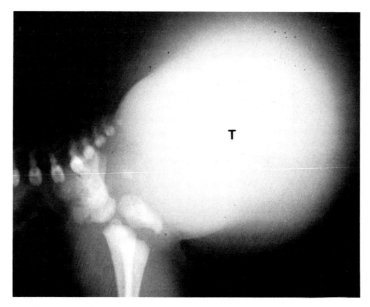

234. Radiograph of same neonate after birth: (T) cystic teratoma arising from lower sacral area.

Sacrococcygeal Teratoma (*contd.*)

This extremely rare tumor occurs in 1 of 40,000 births. It is more common in twins and in girls. It is composed of all three germinal layers; 33% of cases are malignant, and these are usually solid lesions. The majority are benign, and are cystic or mixed, containing small calcified foci.

Figures 233 and 234 illustrate a benign sacrococcygeal teratoma, which appears as a fluid-filled sac (T) projecting from the fetal rump and causing little deformity of the sacrum.

Associated findings are polyhydramnios and, rarely, fetal hydrops.

Twin–Twin Transfusion Syndrome

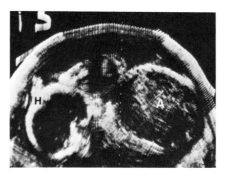

235. Transverse scan of the uterus: (H) small head of the donor twin; (A) large abdomen of the recipient twin.

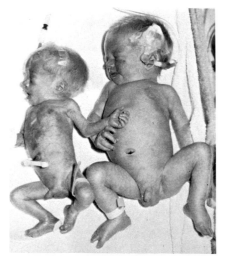

236. Picture of the twins shortly after birth. The donor twin is smaller. The recipient twin is larger.

Twin–twin transfusion syndrome, which occurs in monozygotic twins, is due to shunting of blood through placental arteriovenous anastomoses, and this affects the growth of both fetuses. Sonographic findings include the following:

1. Discrepancy in size between the twins. The donor twin is smaller than the recipient.
2. Hydramnios is often present in the recipient's gestational sac.
3. A single placenta with two umbilical cords. The donor twin may have a two-vessel cord.
4. Hydropic changes in the recipient twin.

Fetal Death

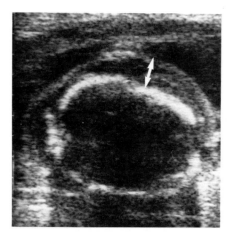

237. Axial scan of fetal head several days after death: (*arrow*) marked subcutaneous edema.

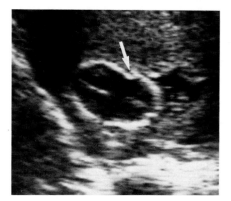

238. Spalding's sign; axial scan of fetal head at 19 weeks of gestation: (*arrow*) overlap of frontal and parietal bones of cranial vault. [*Note.* Dolicocephalic shape of head (i.e., compressed width and elongated occipitofrontal diameter).]

Ultrasound findings are as follows:

Always.   Absent fetal cardiac activity and absent fetal movement.

Less frequent.   Overlapping of skull bones (Spalding's sign); gross distortion of fetal anatomy due to maceration; soft tissue edema greater than 5 mm.

Not commonly visualized.   Thrombus in fetal heart or vascular structures; gas in fetal heart or vascular structures.

Fetal Death (*contd.*)

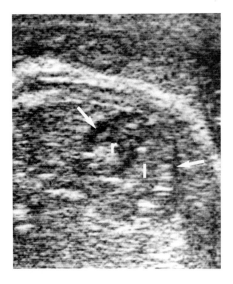

239. Axial scan of fetal chest: (r) right ventricle filled with echogenic clotted blood; (l) left ventricle filled with echogenic clotted blood; (*arrows*) hypoechoic ventricular walls.

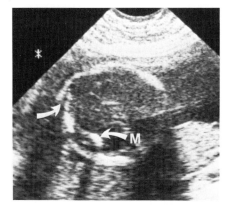

240. Pseudo-Spalding's sign; axial scan of normal fetal head at 26 weeks of gestation: (*arrow*) apparent overlap of fetal bones in an ultrasound artifact; (M) pseudomass inside fetal head due to echoes arising from normally ossified petrous ridge.

Chapter 11

FETAL MEASUREMENTS AND CALCULATIONS

Dating of Pregnancy

Weeks of gestation	Preferred dating measurement	Approximate accuracy
3-5	None	
5-6	Gestational sac diameter	±1 Week
6-12	Crown-rump length	±3-7 Days
12-20	1. Biparietal diameter	±1 Week
	2. Femur	±1 Week
20-30	1. Biparietal diameter	±2 Weeks
	2. Femur	±2 Weeks
	3. Abdominal circumference	±3 Weeks
30-40	1. Biparietal diameter	±3.5 Weeks
	2. Femur	±4 Weeks
	3. Abdominal circumference	±4 Weeks

Rules of Thumb for Calculating Gestational Age

The fetal parameters most commonly used to predict gestational age (GA) are the crown–rump length (CRL), the biparietal diameter (BPD), and femur length (FL). The appropriate tables are found in the Appendix; however, approximate formulas or rules of thumb may be used to calculate quickly gestational age without reference to tables or computers.

Crown–rump length: GA (weeks) = CRL (cm) + 6.5

Biparietal diameter:

GA (weeks) = 4 × BPD (cm)   for   BPD of 6 to 9 cm

GA (weeks) = 4 × BPD (cm) + correction   for   BPD of 2 to 5 cm

BPD (cm):	2	3	4	5	6	7	8	9
Factor:	×4	×4	×4	×4	×4	×4	×4	×4
Correction:	+5	+3	+2	+1				
GA (weeks):	13	15	18	21	24	28	32	36

Femur length:

GA (weeks) = 5 × FL (cm)   for   FL of 7 to 8 cm

GA (weeks) = 5 × FL (cm) + correction   for   FL of 2 to 6 cm

Femur (cm):	2	3	4	5	6	7	8
Factor:	×5	×5	×5	×5	×5	×5	×5
Correction:	+6	+4	+3	+2	+1		
GA (weeks):	16	19	23	27	31	35	40

Fetal Head

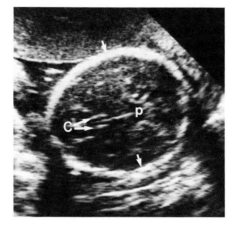

241. Axial scan of fetal head (sector scanner): (*arrows*) points demarcating the biparietal diameter; (C) cavum septi pellucidi; (P) cerebral peduncles.

From 12 weeks to full term, the axial scan of the fetal head may be used to estimate the gestational age. The axial scan should contain the cavum septi pellucidi (in the anterior portion of brain) and the cerebral peduncles or thalami (in the midposterior portion of the brain). The head shape should be oval, and the midline echo from the interhemispheric fissure should be in the midline. The biparietal diameter (BPD) is measured from the outer edge of the near surface to the inner edge of the far surface. The occipitofrontal diameter (OFD) is measured from the midpoint of the occipital bone to the midpoint of the frontal bone. The BPD predicts the menstrual age with the following approximate uncertainty ranges:

12 to 20 weeks, ± 1 week;
20 to 30 weeks, ± 2 weeks;
30 to 40 weeks, ± 3.5 weeks.

Fetal Head (*contd.*)

The main use for the OFD is to calculate the cephalic index (BPD/OFD) and/or the corrected BPD:

$$\text{Corrected BPD} = [(\text{BPD} \times \text{OFD})/1.265]^{1/2}$$

The normal range of cephalic index is 0.75–0.83. In practice, the corrected BPD is more useful because this can be used to estimate gestational age directly. The corrected BPD is useful when there is molding of the fetal head causing dolicocephaly: The BPD is smaller than expected and the OFD larger than expected.

The head circumference is not commonly used to estimate gestational age; however, the ratio of head circumference to abdominal circumference (HC/AC) can be useful in detecting asymmetric growth retardation. To calculate the head circumference, we measure the BPD (O–O) (outer edge to outer edge) and the OFD (O–O) (outer edge to outer edge):

$$\text{HC} = \pi \times \tfrac{1}{2}[\text{BPD(O–O)} + \text{OFD(O–O)}]$$

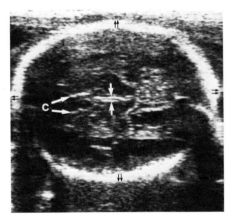

242. Axial scan of fetal head (linear array scanner): (C) cavum septi pellucidi; (*white arrows*) walls of third ventricle; (*black arrows*) points demarcating the BPD (O–O) and OFD (O–O).

Fetal Abdomen

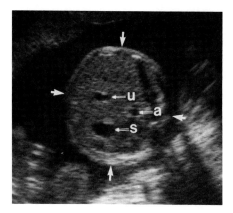

243. Axial scan of fetal abdomen: (U) umbilical portion of left portal vein inside fetal liver; (A) aorta; (S) stomach; (*arrows*) points from which the abdominal diameters are measured.

The circumference of the fetal abdomen is useful in estimating fetal weight. An axial scan of the fetal abdomen is obtained perpendicular to the long axis of the fetal spine. The scan is through fetal liver, and it should contain the umbilical portion of the left portal vein. If the entire length of the umbilical vein within the fetal abdomen is visualized, then the scan is not a true axial scan and thus is not suitable for measuring the abdominal circumference. The circumference may be measured directly by using a map reader or, more conveniently, by measuring the external orthogonal diameters and then using the approximation formula:

$$\text{Circumference} = \pi \times \tfrac{1}{2}(D_1 + D_2)$$

The abdominal circumference may also be used for dating purposes, but it is less accurate than the biparietal diameter or femur length. The main use for abdominal circumference is calculation of fetal weights.

Fetal Femur

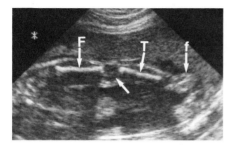

244. Long-axis scan of fetal leg: (F) femur; (T) tibia; (f) foot; (K) knee epiphyses. No evidence of ossification within distal femoral nor proximal tibial epiphyses. Note through-transmission behind knee.

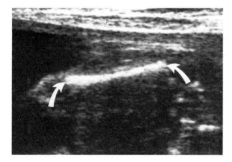

245. Sagittal scan of fetal femur: (*arrows*) measurement points for femur length. These points represent the ends of the ossified portion of the femoral diaphysis.

The femur length should be measured in a sagittal plane where the ossified portion of the diaphysis appears as a hyperechoic, straight structure. In a coronal scan plane, the femur appears slightly curved because of the shape of the femur. An accurate femur length will predict menstrual age with similar accuracy compared to the biparietal diameter (BPD). However, we find that accurate measurements of femur length are more difficult than BPD and therefore less reliable in predicting menstrual age than BPD. Inaccuracies arise for the following reasons:

1. When the true long axis is not obtained, the length is underestimated. There are no landmarks to indicate when the scan includes the true long axis.

2. Ultrasound machines are better calibrated and more accurate in determining axial lengths (i.e., in the direction parallel to the beam) than horizontal lengths (i.e., in the direction perpendicular to the beam).

3. The accuracy of horizontal measurements varies with depth.

4. When the femur is obliquely oriented, measurement is more difficult and less accurate.

5. Leg motion may cause difficulty in obtaining measurements.

Assessment of Fetal Growth

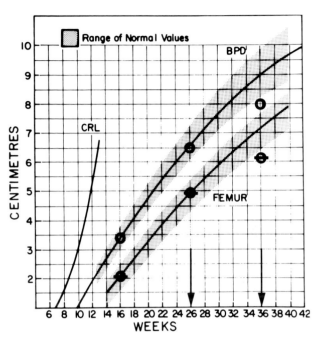

246. Graphs of crown–rump length (CRL), biparietal diameter (BPD), and femur length (FL): (VS) gestational age; (O) BPD values at 16, 26, and 36 weeks of gestation; (O) FL values at 16, 26, and 36 weeks of gestation; (*arrows*) weeks of gestation based on the initial study where the BPD and FL indicated 16 weeks of gestation. The values for BPD and FL in the second and third studies were plotted along the vertical axes corresponding to 26 and 36 weeks of gestation.

A sonogram in early pregnancy (e.g., approximately 16 weeks) allows accurate determination of dates by measuring the BPD and FL (Fig. 246). Scans later in pregnancy can then accurately assess the growth in BPD and FL. For example, a scan performed 10 weeks later would be plotted as follows: The gestational age is now 16 + 10, or 26 weeks, which is marked on the horizontal axis. The BPD and FL are plotted along the vertical line corresponding to 26 weeks and compared to the normal values of the curve. In this example, the BPD and FL have grown the expected amount.

For another scan performed 10 weeks after the second scan (i.e., at 36 weeks), the measured BPD and FL are plotted along the vertical line corresponding to 36 weeks. In this example, the growth for BPD and FL is below normal limits.

Estimated Fetal Weight

When the menstrual age of the pregnancy is known, then an estimated fetal weight in the third trimester can provide valuable information to the attending physician.

Total intrauterine volume may be measured, but this is less accurate and not possible when using real-time equipment only.

Fetal weight may be estimated by using formulas or tables that require one of the following set of fetal measurements: (a) biparietal diameter (BPD) and abdominal circumference; (b) BPD, femur length, and abdominal circumference; and (c) femur length and abdominal circumference. The formulas are given in the Appendix. These formulas will predict fetal weight with an error range of approximately ±15%.

Intrauterine Growth Retardation

The most common indication for estimating fetal weight is for suspected intrauterine growth retardation (IUGR). The information is useful in deciding whether or not delivery is advisable. Growth retardation is present if the weight is below the third percentile for the number of weeks of gestation. If the gestational age is not known, then the estimated fetal weight is much less useful, because it is impossible to assign the weight to a percentile of fetal weight.

IUGR may be the symmetric type, where the head and body are equally affected [the ratio of head circumference/abdominal circumference (HC/AC) is normal], or the asymmetric type, where the head is less affected than the body (the HA/AC is high). Symmetric IUGR, the less common type, may be due to familial small size, intrauterine infections, or chromosomal abnormalities associated with reduced growth potential. Asymmetric IUGR, the more common type, is usually due to poor placental perfusion. Decreased placental perfusion is often due to maternal diseases that cause vascular damage in the uteroplacental circulation (e.g., diabetes mellitus, chronic hypertension, renal diseases, and some autoimmune diseases, such as lupus erythematosus). Placental perfusion may also be impaired by primary placental pathology, such as placental infarcts.

In symmetric IUGR, the fetal measurements are low throughout pregnancy. In asymmetric IUGR, the fetal abdominal and head measurements are normal in early pregnancy, but growth decreases in the third trimester. (See *Assessment of Fetal Growth*, p. 167.)

Appendix

Gestational Age Derived from Crown–Rump Length

Crown-rump length (mm)	Gestational age[a] (weeks)	Crown-rump length (mm)	Gestational age (weeks)	Crown-rump length (mm)	Gestational age (weeks)
5	6.0	24	9.0	43	10.9
6	6.2	25	9.1	44	11.0
7	6.4	26	9.3	45	11.1
8	6.6	27	9.4	46	11.2
9	6.8	28	9.5	47	11.3
10	7.0	29	9.6	48	11.4
11	7.2	30	9.7	49	11.4
12	7.4	31	9.8	50	11.5
13	7.5	32	9.9	51	11.6
14	7.7	33	10.0	52	11.7
15	7.8	34	10.1	53	11.8
16	8.0	35	10.2	54	11.8
17	8.1	36	10.3	55	11.9
18	8.3	37	10.4	56	12.0
19	8.4	38	10.5	57	12.1
20	8.5	39	10.6	58	12.2
21	8.7	40	10.7	59	12.2
22	8.8	41	10.8	60	12.3
23	8.9	42	10.8		

Data were derived from the following equation using the computer programs enclosed:

$$GA = (8.052 \times CRL^{1/2} + 23.73)/7$$

where GA is gestational age, and CRL is crown-rump length. (From Robinson HP, Fleming JEE. A critical evaluation of sonar "crown-rump length" measurements. *Br J Obstet Gynecol* 1975;82:702-10.)

[a]The crown-rump length predicts the gestational age within the following approximate range: ±5 days.

Gestational Age Derived from Biparietal Diameter

Biparietal diameter (mm)	Gestational age[a] (weeks)	Biparietal diameter (mm)	Gestational age (weeks)	Biparietal diameter (mm)	Gestational age (weeks)
15	12.1	44	19.3	73	29.3
16	12.3	45	19.6	74	29.7
17	12.5	46	19.9	75	30.1
18	12.8	47	20.2	76	30.5
19	13.0	48	20.5	77	30.9
20	13.2	49	20.8	78	31.3
21	13.4	50	21.1	79	31.7
22	13.6	51	21.5	80	32.1
23	13.8	52	21.8	81	32.5
24	14.1	53	22.1	82	33.0
25	14.3	54	22.4	83	33.4
26	14.5	55	22.8	84	33.8
27	14.8	56	23.1	85	34.2
28	15.0	57	23.4	86	34.7
29	15.2	58	23.8	87	35.1
30	15.5	59	24.1	88	35.6
31	15.7	60	24.5	89	36.0
32	16.0	61	24.8	90	36.5
33	16.3	62	25.2	91	36.9
34	16.5	63	25.5	92	37.4
35	16.8	64	25.9	93	37.8
36	17.0	65	26.3	94	38.3
37	17.3	66	26.6	95	38.7
38	17.6	67	27.0	96	39.2
39	17.9	68	27.4	97	39.7
40	18.1	69	27.7	98	40.2
41	18.4	70	28.1	99	40.6
42	18.7	71	28.5	100	41.1
43	19.0	72	28.9	101	41.6
				102	42.1

Data were derived from the following equation using the computer programs enclosed:

$$GA = 9.54 + 0.1482 \times BPD + 0.001676 \times BPD^2$$

where GA is gestational age, and BPD is biparietal diameter. (From Hadlock FP, Deter RL, Harrist RB, Park SK. Estimating fetal age: computer-assisted analysis of multiple fetal growth parameters. *Radiology* 1984;152:497–501.)

[a]The biparietal diameter predicts the gestational age within the following approximate ranges: for 12 to 20 weeks, ±1 week; for 20 to 30 weeks, ± 2 weeks; for 30 to 40 weeks, ±3.5 weeks.

Gestational Age Derived from Femur Length

Femur length (mm)	Gestational age[a] (weeks)	Femur length (mm)	Gestational age (weeks)	Femur length (mm)	Gestational age (weeks)
8	12.0	34	20.9	60	31.1
9	12.3	35	21.2	61	31.6
10	12.6	36	21.6	62	32.0
11	12.9	37	22.0	63	32.4
12	13.3	38	22.4	64	32.9
13	13.6	39	22.7	65	33.3
14	13.9	40	23.1	66	33.7
15	14.2	41	23.5	67	34.2
16	14.6	42	23.9	68	34.6
17	14.9	43	24.3	69	35.0
18	15.2	44	24.7	70	35.5
19	15.6	45	25.0	71	35.9
20	15.9	46	25.4	72	36.4
21	16.3	47	25.8	73	36.8
22	16.6	48	26.2	74	37.3
23	16.9	49	26.6	75	37.7
24	17.3	50	27.0	76	38.2
25	17.6	51	27.4	77	38.6
26	18.0	52	27.8	78	39.1
27	18.3	53	28.2	79	39.5
28	18.7	54	28.6	80	40.0
29	19.0	55	29.1	81	40.5
30	19.4	56	29.5	82	40.9
31	19.8	57	29.9	83	41.4
32	20.1	58	30.3	84	41.9
33	20.5	59	30.7		

Data were derived from the following equation using the computer programs enclosed:

$$GA = 9.5411757 + 0.2977451 \times FL + 0.0010388013 \times FL^2$$

where GA is gestational age, and FL is femur length. (From Jeanty P, Rodesch F, Delbeke D, Dumont JE. Estimation of gestational age from measurements of fetal long bones. *J Ultrasound Med* 1984;3:75–9.)

[a]The femur length predicts the gestational age within the following approximate ranges: for 12 to 20 weeks, ±1 week; for 20 to 30 weeks, ±2 weeks; for 30 to 40 weeks, ±4 weeks.

Ratio of Head Circumference to Abdominal Circumference as a Function of Gestational Age

Gestational age (weeks)	HC/AC[a]	Gestational age (weeks)	HC/AC	Gestational age (weeks)	HC/AC
22	1.14	29	1.08	36	1.02
23	1.13	30	1.07	37	1.01
24	1.12	31	1.06	38	1.00
25	1.11	32	1.05	39	0.99
26	1.10	33	1.04	40	0.99
27	1.09	34	1.04	41	0.98
28	1.09	35	1.03	42	0.97

Data were derived from the following equation using the computer programs enclosed:

$$HC/AC = 1.32293 - 0.0084471 \times MA$$

where MA is menstrual age, and HC/AC is ratio of head circumference to abdominal circumference. (From Deter RL, Hadlock FP, Harrist RB. Evaluation of normal fetal growth and the detection of intrauterine growth retardation. In Cullen PW, ed, *Ultrasonography in obstetrics and gynecology.* Philadelphia: WB Saunders, 1983:137.)

[a]The range of normal HC/AC ratios is approximately ±0.1 (±2 SD).

Ratio of Femur Length to Abdominal Circumference as a Function of Gestational Age

After 20 weeks of gestation, the value of the ratio of femur length to abdominal circumference (FL/AC) is a constant. The mean is 22.0 with a range of ±2.2 (±2 SD). Suspect intrauterine growth retardation (IUGR) when FL/AC is greater than 24.0, and suspect macrosomia when FL/AC is less than 20.5.

Estimated Fetal Weight (in Grams)

BPD (cm)	Abdominal Circumference (cm)										
	20	22	24	26	28	30	32	34	36	38	40
6.0	706	811	932	1,071	1,231	1,414	1,624	1,866	2,144	2,463	2,829
6.2	744	853	977	1,120	1,284	1,471	1,686	1,932	2,215	2,538	2,909
6.4	784	896	1,025	1,171	1,339	1,531	1,751	2,001	2,288	2,616	2,991
6.6	826	942	1,074	1,225	1,397	1,594	1,817	2,073	2,364	2,696	3,075
6.8	870	990	1,126	1,281	1,458	1,658	1,887	2,147	2,442	2,778	3,161
7.0	916	1,040	1,181	1,340	1,521	1,726	1,959	2,223	2,523	2,863	3,250
7.2	965	1,093	1,238	1,401	1,586	1,796	2,044	2,302	2,607	2,951	3,341
7.4	1,017	1,149	1,297	1,465	1,655	1,869	2,111	2,384	2,693	3,041	3,435
7.6	1,072	1,207	1,360	1,533	1,727	1,945	2,192	2,469	2,782	3,134	3,531
7.8	1,129	1,269	1,426	1,603	1,801	2,025	2,275	2,557	2,874	3,230	3,631
8.0	1,189	1,333	1,495	1,676	1,879	2,107	2,362	2,649	2,969	3,329	3,733
8.2	1,253	1,401	1,567	1,753	1,960	2,193	2,462	2,743	3,068	3,431	3,838
8.4	1,320	1,473	1,643	1,833	2,045	2,282	2,546	2,841	3,169	3,536	3,945
8.6	1,390	1,548	1,722	1,917	2,134	2,375	2,643	2,942	3,274	3,644	4,056
8.8	1,465	1,626	1,806	2,005	2,226	2,472	2,744	3,047	3,383	3,756	4,170
9.0	1,543	1,709	1,893	2,097	2,322	2,572	2,849	3,155	3,495	3,871	4,287
9.2	1,626	1,796	1,984	2,193	2,423	2,677	2,958	3,268	3,611	3,989	4,408
9.4	1,712	1,887	2,080	2,293	2,527	2,786	3,070	3,384	3,738	4,111	4,536
9.6	1,804	1,984	2,181	2,398	2,637	2,899	3,188	3,505	3,854	4,237	4,659
9.8	1,900	2,085	2,286	2,508	2,751	3,017	3,309	3,630	3,981	4,367	4,790
10.0	2,002	2,191	2,397	2,623	2,870	3,140	3,436	3,759	4,113	4,501	4,924

[a]Data were derived from the following equation using the computer programs enclosed:

$$\log_{10} Wt = 1.335 - 0.000034 \times AC \times FL + 0.00316 \times BPD + 0.00457 \times AC + 0.01623 \times FL$$

where Wt is fetal weight (grams), AC is abdominal circumference, FL is femur length, BCD is biparietal diameter. From Shepard MJ, Richards VA, Berkowitz RL, Warsof SL, Hobbins JC. An evaluation of two equations for predicting fetal weight by ultrasound. *Am J Obstet Gynecol* 1982;141:47–54.
The above formula will predict fetal weight with an error range of approximately ±15%.

Normal Fetal Weight

Gestational age (weeks)	Fetal weight (g), mean	10th-90th Percentile
28	1,200	(750-1,700)
29	1,325	(875-1,900)
30	1,500	(1,000-2,100)
31	1,660	(1,150-2,300)
32	1,850	(1,300-2,500)
33	2,000	(1,500-2,700)
34	2,200	(1,700-2,900)
35	2,400	(1,900-3,100)
36	2,600	(2,100-3,300)
37	2,800	(2,300-3,450)
38	3,000	(2,500-3,600)
39	3,170	(2,670-3,770)
40	3,400	(2,750-3,900)
41	3,450	(2,800-4,000)
42	3,420	(2,850-4,060)

Data were derived from a graph in Brenner WE, Edelman DA, Hendricks CH. A standard of fetal growth for the United States of America. *Am J Obstet Gynecol* 1976;126:555.

Summary of Obstetric Calculation Package and Computer Programs for a Pocket Computer

Program No.	Program name[a]	Input variables[a]	Input units	Output units	Reference[b]
P1	GA from LMP and date	Day, month (LMP) Day, month (present date)	Numerals	Weeks	
P2	GA from CRL	CRL	mm	Weeks	Robinson and Fleming (1975)
P3	GA from BPD	BDP	mm	Weeks	Hadlock et al. (1984)
P4	GA from FL	FL	mm	Weeks	Jeanty et al. (1984)
P5	GA from AC	D1, D2	mm	Weeks	Hadlock et al. (1982)
P6	Fetal weight	BPD, D1, D2	mm	grams	Shepard et al. (1982)
P7	Fetal weight	BPD, D1, D2, FL	mm	grams	Hadlock et al. (1985)
P8	Fetal weight	D1, D2, FL	Weeks	grams	Hadlock et al. (1985)
P9	Ideal weights	GA	Weeks	grams	Greenes (1982)
P10	BPD corrected	BDP, OFD	mm	mm	Doubilet and Greenes (1984)
P11	Ideal BPD	GA	Weeks	mm	Jeanty et al. (1984)
P12	HC/AC ratio (calculated)	BPD (O-O), OFD (O-O), D1, D2	mm	Ratio	
P13	HC/AC (from GA)	GA	Weeks	Ratio	Deter et al. (1983)
P14	FL/AC (calculated)	FL, D1, D2	mm	Ratio	Hadlock et al. (1985)
P15	No. of weeks between two dates		Dates	Weeks	Radioshack, owner's manual

Designed for Radioshack TRS-80 pocket computer model PC-3. The program can generate a brief written record of the calculated results on an attached printer, or the pocket computer can function without the attached printer.

[a](GA) gestational age; (CRL) crown–rump length; (BPD) biparietal diameter; (OFD) occipitofrontal diameter; (FL) femur length; (D1) abdominal diameter 1; (D2) abdominal diameter 2 (orthogonal to 1); (LMP) last menstrual period; (HC) head circumference; (AC) abdominal circumference.

[b]Programs are based on equations appearing in the listed references. (See specific program for complete reference.)

P1 Gestational Age from Last Menstrual Period and Present Date

Formula

GA = [number of present day (of 365)

− number of LMP day (of 365)]/7

Computer Program

```
10  "A" : INPUT "LMP DAY = ";A
12  INPUT "LMP MONTH = ";B
14  INPUT "PRESENT DAY = ";C
16  INPUT "PRESENT MONTH = ";D
20  M = A + 30.5 * B
22  N = C + 30.5 * D
24  W = (N-M)/7
25  W = (INT (W * 10 + .5))/10
26  X = (N-M + 365)/7
27  X = (INT (X * 10 + .5))/10
28  IF W>0 THEN 34
30  IF W<0 THEN 32
32  PRINT "LMP AGE = ";X;" WKS"
33  LPRINT "LMP AGE = ";X;" WKS"
34  PRINT "LMP AGE = ";W;" WKS"
35  LPRINT "LMP AGE = ";W;" WKS"
```

P2 Gestational Age from Crown–Rump Length

Reference

Robinson HP, Fleming JEE. A critical evaluation of sonar "crown–rump length" measurements. *Br J Obstet Gynecol* 1975;82:702–10.

Formula
GA = [8.052(CRL)$^{1/2}$ + 23.73]/7

Computer Program

```
40  "S" : INPUT "CRL(MM) = ";C
42  A = (8.052 * SQRC + 23.73)/7
43  A = (INT (A * 10 + .5))/10
45  PRINT "CRL AGE = ";A;" WKS"
46  LPRINT "CRL = ";C;" MM"
47  LPRINT "CRL AGE = ";A;" WKS"
```

P3 Gestational Age from Biparietal Diameter

Reference

Hadlock FP, Deter RL, Harrist RB, Park SK. Estimating fetal age: computer-assisted analysis of multiple fetal growth parameters. *Radiology* 1984;152: 497–501.

Formula

$$GA = 9.54 + \frac{1.482}{10}BPD + \frac{0.1676}{100}(BPD)^2$$

Computer Program

```
50   "D":INPUT "BPD(MM) = ";B
52   A = 9.54 + .1482 * B + .001676 * B^2
54   A = (INT (A * 10 + .5))/10
56   PRINT "BPD AGE = ";A;" WKS"
58   LPRINT "BPD = ";B;" MM"
59   LPRINT "BPD AGE = ";A;" WKS"
```

P4 Gestational Age from Femur Length

Reference

Jeanty P, Rodesch F, Delbeke D, Dumont JE. Estimation of gestational age from measurements of fetal long bones. *J Ultrasound Med* 1984;3:75–9.

Formula

$$GA = 9.5411757 + 0.2977451\ FL + 0.0010388013(FL)^2$$

Computer Program

```
60   "F" : INPUT "FEM(MM) = ";F
62   A = 9.5411757 + .297745 * F + .0010388013 * F^2
64   A = (INT (A * 10 + .5))/10
66   PRINT "FL AGE = ";A;" WKS"
68   LPRINT "FL = ";F;" MM"
69   LPRINT "FL AGE = ";A;" WKS"
```

P5 Gestational Age from Abdominal Diameter

Reference

Hadlock FP, Deter RL, Harrist RB, et al. Fetal abdominal circumference as a predictor of menstrual age. *Am J Roentgenol* 1982;139:367–70.

Reference

$$GA = 7.6070 + 0.7645 \ AC + 0.00393(AC)^2$$

Computer Program

```
70  "G" : INPUT "AD1(MM) = ";D
71  INPUT "AD2(MM) = ";E
72  F = π*(D+E)/20
74  A = 7.6070 + 0.7645*F + 0.00393*^2
75  A = (INT (A * 10 + .5))/10
76  PRINT "AC AGE = ";A;" WKS"
77  LPRINT "AD1 = ";D;" MM"
78  LPRINT "AD2 = ";E;" MM"
79  LPRINT "AC AGE = ";A;" WKS"
```

P6 Estimated Fetal Weight from Biparietal Diameter and Abdominal Diameters

Reference

Shepard MJ, Richards VA, Berkowitz RL, Warsof SL, Hobbins JC. An evaluation of two equations for predicting fetal weight by ultrasound. *Am J Obstet Gynecol* 1982;141:47–54.

Formula

$$\log_{10} Wt = -1.7492 + 0.166 \ BPD + 0.046 \ AC - 2.646 \ (AC \times BPD)/1,000$$

P6 Estimated Fetal Weight from Biparietal Diameter and Abdominal Diameter (*contd.*)

Computer Program

```
80   "H" : INPUT "BPD(MM) = ";B
82   INPUT "AD1(MM) = ";D
84   INPUT "AD2(MM) = ";E
86   Z = −1.7492 + .0166 * B + .0046 * (D+E)/2*π
        −.02646 * (D+E)/2 * π * B * .001
88   W = 10^(3+Z)
90   W = INT (W + .5)
91   PRINT "WT(BPD,ABDO) = ";W;" GM"
92   LPRINT "BPD = ";B;" MM"
93   LPRINT "AD1 = ";D;" MM"
94   LPRINT "AD2 = ";E;" MM"
95   LPRINT "WT(BPD,ABDO) = ";W;" GM"
```

P7 Estimated Fetal Weight from Biparietal Diameter, Abdominal Diameters, and Femur Length

Reference

Hadlock FP, Harrist RB, Sharman RS, Deter RL, Park SK. Estimation of fetal weight with the use of head, body, and femur measurements—A prospective study. *Am J Obstet Gynecol* 1985;151:333–7.

Formula

$$\log_{10} Wt = 1.335 - 0.000034\ AC \times FL + 0.00316\ BPD$$
$$+0.00457\ AC + 0.01623\ FL$$

Computer Program

```
100   "J" : INPUT "BPD(MM) = ";B
102   INPUT "AD1(MM) = ";D
104   INPUT "AD2(MM) = ";E
106   INPUT "FL (MM) = ";F
108   C = π * (D+E)/2
110   Z = 1.335 − .000034 * C * F + .00316 * B
          + .00457 * C + .01623 * F
112   W = 10^Z
114   W = INT (W + .5)
115   PRINT "WT(BPD,A,F) = ";W;" GM"
116   LPRINT "WT(BPD,A,F) = ";W;" GM"
```

P8 Estimated Fetal Weight from Abdominal Diameters and Femur Length

Reference

Hadlock FP, Harrist RB, Sharman RS, Deter RL, Park SK. Estimation of fetal weight with the use of head, body, and femur measurements—A prospective study. *Am J Obstet Gynecol* 1985;151:333–7.

Formula

$$\log_{10} Wt = 1.304 + 0.005281\ AC + 0.01938\ FL$$
$$-0.00004\ AC \times FL$$

Computer Program

```
120   "K" : INPUT "AD1(MM) = ";D
122   INPUT "AD2(MM) = ";E
124   INPUT "FL(MM) = ";F
126   C = π * (D+E)/2
128   Z = 1.304 + .005281 * C + .01938 * F
         − .00004 * C * F
130   W = 10^Z
132   W = INT (W + .5)
133   PRINT "WT(FL,ABDO) = ";W;" GM"
134   LPRINT "WT(FL,ABDO) = ";W;" GM"
```

P9 Ideal Fetal Weight from Gestational Age

Reference

Greenes RA. OBUS: A microcomputer system for measurement, calculation, reporting, and retrieval of obstetric ultrasound examinations. *Radiology* 1982;144:879–83.

Formula

$$Wt = -2108.63 + 55.171\ W + 2.084\ W^2$$

Computer Program

```
140   "L" : INPUT "WKS =";A
142   W = −2108.63 + 55.171 * A + 2.084 * A^2
144   W = INT (W + .5)
145   PRINT "AVG WT = ";W;" GM"
146   LPRINT "WEEKS = ";A
147   LPRINT "AVG WT = ";W;" GM"
```

P10   Biparietal Diameter Corrected

Reference

Doubilet PM, Greenes RA. Improved prediction of gestational age from fetal head measurements. *AJR* 1984;142:797–800.

Formula

$BPD' = (BPD \times OFD/1.265)^{1/2}$

Computer Program

```
150    "=" : INPUT "BPD(MM) = ";B
152    INPUT "OFD (MM)= ";O
156    Z = B*O/1.265
157    Y = SQRZ
158    Y = (INT (Y * 10 + .5))/10
159    PRINT "NEW BPD = ";Y;" MM"
160    LPRINT "BPD = ";B;" MM"
161    LPRINT "OFD = ";O;" MM"
162    LPRINT "NEW BPD = ";Y;" MM"
```

P11   Ideal Biparietal Diameter (from Gestational Age)

Reference

Jeanty P, Cousaert E, Hobbins JC, Tuck B, Bracken M, Cantraine F. A longitudinal study of fetal head biometry. *Am J Perinatol* 1984;1:118–28.

Formula

$BPD = -19.634 + 3.0209\ W + 0.042134\ W^2$
$\qquad -0.0011756\ W^3$

Computer Program

```
170    "Z" : INPUT "WKS= ";W
172    B = -19.634 + 3.0209 * W + .042134 * W^2 - .0011756 * W^3
174    B = (INT (B * 10 + .5))/10
175    PRINT "BPD(WKS) = ";B;" MM"
176    LPRINT "WEEKS = ";W
177    LPRINT "BPD(WKS) = ";B;" MM"
```

P12 Ratio of Head Circumference to Abdominal Circumference (Calculated Value)

Formula

$$\frac{HC}{AC} = \frac{BPD(O-O) + OFD(O-O)}{AD1 + AD2}$$

Computer Program

```
180  "X": INPUT "BPD(O-O)(MM) = ";A
182  INPUT "OFD(O-O)(MM) = ";B
184  INPUT "AD1 (MM) = ";C
186  INPUT "AD2 (MM) = ";D
188  E = (A+B)/(C+D)
190  E = (INT (E * 100 + .5))/100
191  PRINT "HC/AC = ";E
192  LPRINT "HC/AC = ";E
```

P13 Ratio of Head Circumference to Abdominal Circumference (from Gestational Age)

Reference

Deter RL, Haddock FP, Harrist RB. Evaluation of normal fetal growth and detection of intrauterine growth retardation. In: Callen PW, ed. *Ultrasonography in obstetrics and gynecology*. Philadelphia: WB Saunders, 1983:137.

Formula

HC/AC = 1.32293 −0.0084471 MA

Computer Program

```
200  "C" : INPUT "GEST AGE (WKS) = ";A
202  B = 1.32293 − .0084471*A
204  B = (INT (B * 100 + .5))/100
205  PRINT "HC/AC(WKS) = ";B;" +−0.1"
206  LPRINT "GEST AGE = ";A;" WKS"
207  LPRINT "HC/AC(WKS) = ";B;" +−0.1"
```

P14   Ratio of Femur Length to Abdominal Circumference (Calculated Value)

Reference

Hadlock FP, Harrist RB, Fearneyhough TC, et al. Use of femur length/abdominal circumference ratio in detecting the macrosomic fetus. *Radiology* 1985;154:503–5.

Formula

$$\frac{FL}{AC} = \frac{FL}{\pi/2(AD1 + AD2)}$$

Computer Program

```
210   "V" : INPUT "FL(MM) = ";A
212   INPUT "AD1(MM) = ";B
214   INPUT "AD2(MM) = ";C
216   D = (B+C)/2
217   D = π*D
218   E = (A/D)*100
220   E = (INT (E * 10 + .5))/10
221   PRINT "FL/AC = ";E;" (22+−2)"
222   LPRINT "FL = ";A;" MM"
223   LPRINT "AD1 = ";B;" AD2 = ";C
224   LPRINT "FL/AC = ";E;" (22+−2)"
```

P15 Number of Weeks Between Two Dates

Reference

Adapted from owner's manual of Radioshack TRS-80, PC-3 pocket computer.

Formula

Program subroutine

Computer Program

```
230   "B"
232   INPUT "START YEAR = "; R, "MONTH = ";S, "DAY = ";T
234   INPUT "END YEAR = "; F, "MONTH = ";V, "DAY = ";W
236   H=R
238   G=S:I=T
240   GOSUB 500
242   J=I
244   H=F
246   G=V:I=W
248   GOSUB 500
249   X=I−J
250   M=X/7
251   M = (INT (M * 10 + .5))/10
252   WAIT : PRINT "WEEKS = ",M
253   LPRINT "WEEKS = ",M
254   GOTO 234
500   IF G−3>=0 LET G=G+1: GOTO 520
510   G=G+13 : H= H−1
520   I = INT (365.25*H) + INT (30.6*G)+I
530   I = I− INT (H/100) + INT (H/400) − 306 − 122: RETURN

600   "Z" : END
```